Advance Praise for

SLEEP IT OFF

"What a great book! Captivating all along! It provides really helpful tips on how to change your sleeping habits for better health and I loved the balance between scientific information and personal stories. I found it especially fascinating to read about the impact of hormones and food intake on our sleep. It is a very inspiring guide from an author who really knows what it is to struggle with sleep. I already know whom I am going to gift this book to!" ~Renee C LeBoeuf, PhD, Emeritus Research Professor of Medicine, University of Washington

"I've read a lot of sleep books! This one is different and helpful in a way that others aren't! Stella Loichot takes you through a complete, science-backed process to understand your own sleep situation and create better habits. It will support you in getting a great night's rest EVERY night, not just an occasional anomaly..." ~Jill Avey, CEO Performance and Leadership Coach

This book is so rich! It is a well of information and inspiration. This guide really delivers on its promise. It is motivational and highly educative, but Ms Loichot keeps it entertaining with great humor and a balance of personal experiences, science, and practical applications. I was drawn in from the start and I believe everyone can find themselves in these pages. A superb way to improve our health!! ~Christine Suter, former Licensed Mental Health Counselor

"If you have been struggling with sleep for any reason, this book is for you! Ms. Loichot covers everything from the causes of sleeplessness, the health implications of not getting enough sleep, and practical solutions that you can start using right away. She effortlessly blends scientific information with anecdotal stories to educate and inspire us to do something about our sleepless nights. Sweet dreams!" ~Elise Kloter, Licensed Massage Therapist

"What's Stella Loichot's secret sauce? It may be a blend of science-based easy explanations, non-judgmental and compassionate perspectives, gentle humor, and a passion for self-discovery and action. Hers are not just words — she walks the talk! We get a glimpse of her personal struggle with sleeping well and the creativity in her approach

to finding a solution. And she helps us realize that having a good night's sleep is not only important but is also within everybody's reach, even if getting there may be outside our comfort zone." ~Osnat Lustig, International Coaching Federation (ICF) Satellite Leader

"Stella Loichot is the best!! She knows how to educate you in a way that really inspires you to make a change for the better. I appreciate her down-to-earth and sustainable approach. A must-read health book for anyone who wants to improve their wellness and reach their body's full potential!!" ~Candice Rose, Corrective Exercise Specialist

SLEEP IT OFF

A Revolutionary Guide to Losing Weight, Beating Diabetes,
and Feeling Your Best Through Optimal Rest

STELLA LOICHOT

Allon-Z Press, Seattle

ISBN 978-1-7356975-0-5 paperback
ISBN 978-1-7356975-1-2 ebook
Library of Congress Control Number: 2020918483
Publisher's Cataloging-in-Publication Data
  Names: Loichot, Stella, author.
  Title: Sleep it off : a revolutionary guide to losing weight , beating diabetes , and feeling your best through optimal rest / Stella Loichot.
  Description: Includes bibliographical references. | Seattle, WA: Allon-Z Press, 2020.
  Identifiers: LCCN: 2020918483 | ISBN: 978-1-7356975-0-5 (pbk.) | 978-1-7356975-1-2 ebook
  Subjects: LCSH Sleep—Health aspects. | Sleep disorders—Treatment. | Insomnia. | BISAC HEALTH & FITNESS / Sleep | BODY, MIND & SPIRIT / Inspiration & Personal Growth
  Classification: LCC RA786 .L65 2020 | DDC 613.7/9—dc23

Illustrations: Salomé Demurger
Interior Design: Rob Siders
Editing: Lola Demurger and Celia Speirs

Printed in the United States of America

Contact the author:
Stella Loichot, NBC-HWC, Allon-Z Coaching, LLC
stella@allonzcoaching.com
Visit: allonZcoaching.com

BEFORE WE START
Who Is This Book For?

This book is for you if you are tired and don't know exactly what to do about it. Perhaps you don't have enough time to sleep, or your sleep is disturbed by others (pets included). Maybe you simply can't fall asleep at night even though you are exhausted, or you wake up in the middle of the night or way too early in the morning. Maybe you actually feel that you sleep just fine, and yet you wake up exhausted with a feeling that sleeping is pointless and not refreshing at all. If you are aware that your sleep is less than optimal, this book is definitely for you.

This book is also for you if you don't feel sleep-deprived but find it hard to lose weight despite sustained efforts; if you struggle with sugar cravings, prediabetes, or type 2 diabetes; or if you are unable to improve your fitness level even though you exercise regularly and vigorously. You might experience recurring injuries, have a weak immune system, feel irritable or depressed, or notice that you are becoming forgetful and have difficulty concentrating. This book is for you if you haven't been feeling your best and have attributed the slowdown to normal wear and tear and aging.

Now, if you are lucky enough to sleep well but are anticipating a big change in your life that might jeopardize your ability to rest, this book will help you be more strategic about your sleep and prepare for unsettling life transitions.

Finally, this book is for you if you want to help someone else who is having issues sleeping or is struggling with weight loss, prediabetes, type 2 diabetes, or fitness. Most adults who have sleep issues fall into one of the following categories:

- People who are obviously tired and deplore their lack of energy during the day. They function well, but only thanks to substantial efforts and many crutches such as coffee, energy drinks, or snacks. They are usually aware of their sleep deprivation and quite vocal about their struggle. They are open to reaching out for help and improving their sleep.

- People who unconsciously compensate for poor sleep with hyperactivity. They are busy and always on the go. If they stop, they crash. I was one of those people. Hormones such as adrenaline, cortisol, and dopamine help them keep up the pace, along with caffeine, snacking, and other coping mechanisms. It is harder for them to realize they have a problem unless they are able to recognize the lesser-known side effects of sleep deprivation.

This practical guide can help both types of people.

WHAT TO EXPECT FROM THIS GUIDE?

This book offers strategies, tips, and a step-by-step approach to help you improve the quality of your sleep. It starts with explaining how sleep works and why your sleep might actually be broken. Then, it will help you assess your current sleep situation and define what changes you could make to be perfectly rested while, at the same time, keeping a lifestyle that works for you and fulfills you. Finally, you will create your own plan of action to improve your sleep and start making improvements right away.

This book is not just for reading. It is a workbook, and you, determined and resourceful reader, will have to do some work. We will use worksheets to help you put together your unique winning sleep plan. Worksheets are included throughout the book so that you can do the work in your book as you read. You will also see examples of how to use the worksheets for best results. I encourage you to download all the worksheets in a convenient ready-to-print workbook. Visit allonzcoaching. com/sleepitoff to download your companion workbook. This is also where you will find additional resources and bonuses to help you improve your sleep even faster.

Do the work as you read, and don't skip any step if you want this process to bring you sustainable results. Go at your own pace. There is no one-size-fits-all solution, but with this guide, you get plenty of tools and a multitude of real-life strategies to select from. Pick the ones that seem the most appealing and suitable for your situation and start experimenting. Don't wait until you have the perfect plan before putting your thoughts into action.

If you find it hard to follow along and implement solutions, feel free to contact me through my website for more resources and personalized support.

WHY DID I WRITE THIS PRACTICAL GUIDE?

I have struggled with my own sleep for decades. At first, I didn't know that I had the power to fix my sleep. Then, I didn't feel like fixing it anymore. And finally, once I was ready to roll up my sleeves and take care of my sleep, I didn't know where to start and how to do it. I wish I'd had a step-by-step system and someone to guide me through the process at that time.

As a practicing Health Coach specializing in Healthy Weight Loss and Diabetes Prevention, I regularly see clients who suffer from sleep deprivation, whether they know it or not. When they come to me for support, it is rarely with the intent to work on their sleep. Some of them have been struggling to lose weight despite the fact that they eat healthily and are physically active. Some of them have reached a plateau in their athletic performance and can't seem to build muscle mass. Some have been recently diagnosed with prediabetes or type 2 diabetes and find it hard to reverse their condition. More often than not, sleep — or lack thereof — is not on their radar.

As soon as our work allows them to identify sleep deprivation as a determining factor in their struggle, they start implementing changes and witness incredible results. I have been so amazed, over the past years, by the impact of sleep on my clients' health and wellness that I have decided to create a guide that could help them and could have helped me when I needed it. I sincerely hope that it will help you, too, to reach optimal wellness and a more fulfilling life.

CONTENTS

INTRODUCTION

As I was writing this book, revealing solutions to the sleep problems I once experienced, I had to dig through my memories to pinpoint where and when the quality of my sleep fell off. I didn't suddenly stop sleeping as often happens to people who experience trauma. The erosion of my sleep took place slowly, over many years, and I didn't realize it. I also didn't realize that I had all the resources within me to turn things around – not only to get better sleep but to lose weight and improve my fitness and overall health.

I used to be a great sleeper – well, as a kid. My princess-style crib was in my parents' room; beyond the comfort of knowing they were close, my dad's gnawing teeth acted like my very own white noise machine. Oddly enough, that same sound would keep me up at night as an adult; we'll get to that soon enough. Even in the daytime, my mom would look for me all over the house and find me in my crib, stealing a nap.

I first started struggling with sleep in high school when stress entered my life for the first time. Besides dating dramas and the quest for independence, I had to work hard to earn straight A's. This involved lots of studying, compounded by pressure to get quality sleep to be sharp the next morning for tests and lectures. The collective stress of school was slowly exacerbated by other s-words that keep many people up at night, including sights, smells, and sounds.

As a people pleaser and rule follower, I would go to bed when instructed – but then would lie there awake, frustrated and stressed out, until everyone else at home went to sleep. The slightest buzz or the smell of a parent's cigarette (it was in the 80s!) would wake me up again. Knowing that was enough to keep me from falling asleep in the first place. My family was very loving and did what they could to be quiet, but who would imagine that touching a light switch was enough to disrupt my sleep?

Things got better when I left for college: no mandatory bedtime and studies were easy. I moved into the basement of a shared house. It was quiet down there, so what little sleep I got was good and it happened on my own terms. As sleep became less of an issue, it also lost its value in my eyes. By the time I started my career in the corporate world, sleep was worth nothing to me. I loved living so much that I felt like bedtime was a forced "time out." I didn't enjoy it at all. I still don't like to sleep today. I'd rather be up all night, reading, playing, working, or gathering with friends to make the world a better place – anything but just lying there, idle, in the dark.

For some, sleep is a sacred bubble, a reward, the satisfying end to a productive day, a chance to unplug and recharge. Ask Fabrice, the love of my life, and he will tell you: there is nothing, nothing at all, that could keep him from sleeping. But that's not me, and that's probably why things turned sour when our kids arrived.

Oh, my children, they are the light of my life, my greatest joy, my heart reborn in human form; and they're also adorable destroyers of sleep! My first kid had no time to "waste" lying down in her crib. Since she did not sleep much, neither did I. I was so nervous about the cardiac jolt that happens when a child's tears make you lurch from a deep sleep that I spent most nights anticipating her cry. My second, born a year later, is much like her father – a sound sleeper – but she loved eating even more than snoozing. She was hungry all the time! So, for three years, I did not once get a full night's sleep. Fabrice, even during his shift on daddy duty, would snore through our babies' cries, so I would tend to them, exhausted and resentful, and more than once on the verge of a nervous breakdown. Sleep deprivation became my new normal. I was in survival mode, like many moms I know. By the time our third child arrived, though, five years after the second, I trusted my gut and went against all the "good parenting recommendations:" we had her sleep in our bed. It made things easier, even if I nursed her for over two years. Something that might seem obvious to many occurred to me in that period: I realized that my decisions could actually affect the quality of my sleep. I didn't have to be a victim; I could somehow shape my sleep the way I wanted. You would think that this awakening (ha!) would be good, right? In fact, it led to my downfall.

Motherhood was my full-time job, but I wanted more. A part-time contract felt like an excellent compromise, and with enough caffeine, days were productive and happy, and the time I spent with my girls was not affected. I had such low standards for sleep quality, the only way I knew I'd missed the mark was being unable to perform at full speed the next day. But soon, a full-time promotion disrupted the equilibrium, and my poor sleep hygiene caught up with me. To make it work, and still be 100% available when my kids were at home, sleep was the first thing to get sacrificed. I awoke at 5 am daily to get two-three hours of work in before the kids woke up. After getting them through the morning routine and off to school, I would head to the office and work until school pickup; then I came home, cooked dinner, helped with homework, got the kids to bed, and collapsed from sheer exhaustion. I also wanted to allocate myself some "me time" in the evening, so, at best, I was getting five hours of sleep per night.

Oddly enough, these were happy years, even though, looking back, I see the flaw in my mindset. At the time, I felt proud that after several years of juggling career and kids, one of my daughters didn't even know I had a full-time job. She thought I was working a few hours per week, which to me, as messed up as it might sound, was proof of success: my job was not affecting my children.

What worried me, though, was that I had little time left in the schedule to be the woman my husband had fallen in love with, three kids, two countries, and all those years ago. He was an avid runner, so I took up running as a hobby, training for 5k and 12k races before upleveling to marathons and triathlons so we could race together. I wanted to "have it all," and for a while, I did. But I could feel deep inside that my fulfillment was fragile and my happiness hanging by a thread. Sleep was the missing link for me to sustain the life I wanted. But I didn't realize it yet.

With the goal of fulfilling my passion and becoming a health coach, I added going back to school to the mix. I managed to hold it all together for a few more months, but then the house of cards fell.

Part of my unconscious attraction to studying nutrition was trying to figure out why I was insidiously gaining weight and not getting fitter, despite all my efforts. My doctors told me that a few extra pounds were nothing to worry about and that it was all part of the aging process. But the uphill trend had me worried. The more I studied, the more I realized my food intake wasn't the problem – it was my lousy sleep diet. All those long hours, all those races, the entertaining, the family trips, the travel abroad… I was running on adrenaline and cortisol, not the mix of rest, nutrition, and self-care that typically powers a body. So even though I was moving through life at an exhilarating pace, my body was being destroyed in the process and I didn't notice. The lack of sleep was central to my overall downward spiral. When it took me months to recover from a cold that had turned into pneumonia, and when one December morning I felt so weak that I couldn't open the garage door to take my daughter to school, I realized that I had hit a wall and was about to lose everything that mattered so much to me. Was it too late to repair the damage?

Fast forward to today. I am still a light sleeper, and with three teens, my own health coaching practice, and aging relatives 5,000 miles away, I would have a few good reasons to be tired and sleep-deprived, but I am not. Why? Because I realized that I have the power to sleep well. I have figured out ways to protect my sleep and make sure I am always rested. I still don't enjoy sleep; that is just not me. But I have made it a priority because now I get it: love it or loathe it, sleep is necessary.

The strategies you'll find in this book did not all come to me in a single moment of enlightenment. The more I learned about what affects sleep, the more I applied things to my life to see what was and was not disrupting my sleep. By trial and error, I learned what could or could not help me sleep better, for longer. The more I worked on this, the more I discovered that I had the power to sleep well. The same can apply to you, too. Not everything you'll read here will work for you, but many of the answers you need are on the pages that follow and can help you improve your sleep in way less time than it took me.

Are you ready to put in the work to optimize your sleep for a better life? Great. Let's begin.

PART I
Awareness

"Knowing is not enough; we must apply."
~Johann Wolfgang von Goethe

Improving your sleep is an adventure. This book will guide you along the journey. The process is simple. It looks like this:

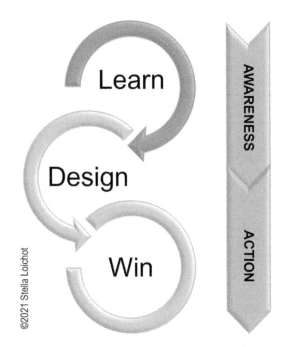

©2021 Stella Loichot

The first part of this book focuses on AWARENESS and will help you become a master of sleep. You will discover the hidden powers of sleep, but also the nuts and bolts of a refreshing night and common obstacles that might get in the way. That's not all! You will also learn everything you need to know about *your* own sleep.

Before we dive in, though, I would like you to briefly reflect on where you are starting from in your sleep journey. Answer the questions on the following page to get a snapshot of your starting point. Of course, you can also write your answers in the ready-to-print companion workbook. Download it for free at allonZcoaching.com/sleepitoff.

Why are you reading this book?

_____

_____

_____

_____

_____

What could be reasons for your poor sleep?

_____

_____

_____

_____

_____

How would better sleep improve your life?

_____

_____

_____

_____

_____

CHAPTER ONE
Hidden Powers of Sleep

"You barely eat anything," said my sister, worried. She was not the only one who had commented on my food intake lately. Even my manager at Allrecipes, where I was working at that time, had noticed. I started wondering whether maybe they were right. I didn't allow myself any treats, I ate way less than anyone around me, and I was back to calorie counting, a weight management technique that I had happily abandoned about 20 years earlier. Yet, despite an average of 13 hours of physical activity per week, that included biking to work and training for a half Ironman, I was gaining weight slowly and consistently. I would have been happy if I had been gaining muscle mass, but that was not the case either. One night, after participating in one of the most beautiful triathlons with my brothers and husband in the French Alps, I was shocked when I saw the pictures my cousin had sent me: my legs and arms were covered with fat I had never noticed before. It finally occurred to me that something was off.

Weight gain wasn't something new and foreign to me. I knew what it was to gain 50 pounds within six months, and it had taken me two decades to figure out healthy and enjoyable ways to keep the pounds under control, despite a less-than-optimal metabolism. This new trend was worrisome and didn't fit in with the otherwise "perfect life" I was living: fast-paced and exhilarating, with my three children, a fulfilling love life, loyal friends, a career I loved, and working toward my nutrition certificate. My schedule was full, but everything was under control, and my life felt like a well-oiled machine. I didn't understand why I couldn't control my weight on top of everything else. Why was it so hard for me to maintain it? What would I have to do to master the way my body handled food? Would I have to eat even less and move even more? That was not possible. I had to find out what I was doing wrong.

I wish I had known then everything I will reveal in this chapter. It would have saved me not just time but a lot of hurt and 18 extra pounds. Here is half-a-life-time's advice from me to you: If you struggle with weight and blood sugar despite all your efforts at eating well and being physically active, sleep is most likely the missing link. What might change your life is understanding not only how sleep affects weight, appetite, body composition, and fitness, but also the way we metabolize sugar and how lack of sleep might lead to diabetes.

Let's dive in!

You probably know that sleep affects our learning process, memory, ability to focus, and even our judgment and capacity to deal with emotions. What you might not know is that blood pressure usually falls during the sleep cycle. Unfortunately, interrupted sleep can hinder this pressure drop, which can lead to hypertension and cardiovascular problems. Research has also shown that insufficient sleep can reduce our body's ability to use insulin, which can lead to the onset of diabetes.[1]

Sleep deprivation can be the root of a variety of problems and a factor in premature death, and yet we keep cutting corners. Many of us end up chronically sleep-deprived but only vaguely aware of it — or completely oblivious! According to the CDC (Centers for Disease Control), more than a third of adults in the U.S. are regularly not getting enough sleep[2], namely 7 to 9 hours per night for most healthy adults, and 7 to 8 hours for older adults[3]. This pattern can be seen on a global level as well, with people in Japan sleeping even less than in any other country of the world, according to *The Economist*.[4]

What I have noticed in my work is that when the consequences of an unhealthy habit are not immediately observable, we don't take them seriously. We don't want to objectively acknowledge the repercussions that our current behavior will have in the distant future, and as a result, we don't try to change. It is not laziness or negligence. It is more that we ignore the negative effects of our lifestyle because we don't suffer from them every day. It is hard to acknowledge that lack of sleep is one culprit responsible for cancers, diabetes, heart disease, and many more disorders. And our feeling of invincibility doesn't go away until we hit a wall or become ill.

What if the effects of sleep deprivation could be more immediate? More tangible and measurable? Knowing that sleep deprivation puts us at risk for gastrointestinal cancer or Alzheimer's disease is not usually enough to make us take action. If we had a better idea of the immediate consequences that shorter nights have on our quality of life, we might be more inclined to take action, prioritize sleep, and implement changes.

What if improving your sleep could help you get stronger and fitter, reduce your sugar cravings to help you lose weight more efficiently, and be your first step toward diabetes prevention or prediabetes reversal?

Of course, sleeping better can also be the missing link to healthy relationships, academic success, or a fulfilling career. This book focuses on the three topics my clients have been struggling with the most: weight loss, blood sugar control, and athletic performance. Brace yourself — the hidden powers of sleep are mind-blowing!

SLEEP AND WEIGHT GAIN

Research shows that sleep deprivation puts people at risk for obesity.[5] A meta-analysis of 18 studies conducted with over 600,000 adults revealed that the risk of obesity was 55% higher for people who slept less than five hours per night.[6] Furthermore, for each additional hour of sleep, people's body mass index (BMI) decreased by 0.35 kg/m^2. Similarly, a study published in the American Journal of Clinical Nutrition confirms that the less we sleep, the more we snack.[7]

At a YMCA Wellness University Conference that I attended in February 2018, one of the speakers was a representative of Jawbone, a seller of wearable fitness trackers and smartphone applications. She presented a study carried out by Jawbone which analyzed data from thousands of users and concluded that the later we go to bed, the more calories we consume the next day. More precisely, the study stated that going to bed 30 minutes earlier at night was linked to eating 50 fewer calories the next day. Looking at it from a weight-loss perspective, going to bed 30 minutes earlier every night could help you lose five pounds over the course of a year, without making any other changes. Thirty extra minutes of sleep were also linked to differences in the kinds of food eaten, depending on how late people went to bed at night. According to Jawbone's report, when we go to bed earlier, we eat healthier foods the next day!

This data was based on fitness accessories, which are not the most accurate source of information, so I encourage readers to take this information with a grain of salt. Yet it remains a useful illustration of the impact of sleep on our weight management efforts. Let's review a few of the reasons sleep deprivation can lead to weight gain and why a regular good night's sleep might help curb our appetite and reduce our weight.

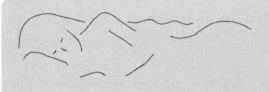

STORYTIME

For many years, Lisa struggled with evening snacking. She was eating mostly healthy foods and cooking homemade dinner at night, but bedtime snacks were out of control. She was extremely frustrated. She felt strong and disciplined all day long, but as soon as the sun went down, her cravings were irresistible. It made it impossible to lose weight, and she was worried that soon her health would suffer and she would not be able to stick around to see her grandchildren become young adults.

To reach her goal of losing 50 pounds, she had to address the snack issue head-on. She knew it but had not been successful so far. Together, we looked at what was really happening at night. To relax after a busy and productive day, Lisa would always settle in front of the TV for three or four hours, and she would invariably end up grabbing cookies, coated nuts, or a candy bar. She had tried very hard to resist the temptation. She would "do good" for a few days, then bounce back to her snacking routine. She had tried to eat healthy snacks instead of treats, but nothing worked: chocolate always won over the celery sticks! We decided to take our attention away from the snacking itself and rather concentrate on everything else she was doing around bedtime. Lisa made the following plan: instead of watching TV, she would first take a warm relaxing bath and then go to bed with a book. She would try for two weeks.

Here is what happened: instead of watching TV for several hours and eating treats every night, she read for about one hour and fell asleep systematically before having time to grab or even think about grabbing a night snack. She ended up skipping her treats easily, without willpower or effort, because she was sleeping. She realized that she did not really miss watching TV. All she needed at night was a way to unwind. With the new routine of reading a book in bed, she ended up sleeping more and eating less. She started working out as a result and lost 23 pounds within a few months, without feeling deprived, which was key to her long-term success. And she felt happier overall. Reading books was something she used to do at a younger age. It gave her joy that she had long forgone and brought back cherished memories.

When You Sleep, You Don't Eat

One reason weight management is easier when we sleep well is that when we sleep more, we spend less time awake, and we don't get as many opportunities to eat. Though this may seem obvious, it is something that most people don't realize, but it can affect weight management significantly.

Lack of Sleep Leads to Poor Choices

Another way sleep affects our weight is that when we are sleep-deprived, we make fewer healthy choices throughout the day.

According to a Berkeley and Harvard study, when we don't sleep well or enough, the areas of our brain that trigger emotions are 60% more active than when we are well-rested.[8] When we are sleep-deprived, we get highly emotional, and this leads to emotional eating. Emotional eating is one of the toughest habits to break for people who are trying to lose weight. Though lack of sleep is not the only reason for emotional eating, it will feed and worsen this habit.

Sleepiness Affects Sugar Cravings

When we feel tired, we look for the quickest and most accessible source of energy available. Usually, that is carbohydrates with a high glycemic index (G.I.), in other words, processed and sugary foods that raise our blood sugar level quickly. Our brain's fuel is glucose, and we get glucose from eating carbohydrates. Foods such as chips, bread, cookies, or an energy bar are the quickest-metabolized source of energy. Our body processes them quickly and brings glucose to our brain faster than if we ate carbohydrates from whole foods. Whole foods are foods that have been minimally processed and refined and don't contain any artificial additives or preservatives. These foods are similar to what they look like in nature. Brown rice, beans, quinoa, fruits, and vegetables are all excellent examples of plant-based whole foods. When we are tired, we naturally and unconsciously go for foods high in processed carbohydrates because our sleepy brain knows that we will get energy right away.

Although a sugary snack or beverage provides the needed sugar rush, it is short-lived and leaves us feeling sluggish and even more exhausted. This leads to our reaching out for yet another sugary snack. The cycle can go on for a long time. The graph on the following page gives an idea of what happens.

Please note that the diagrams in this book are not to scale. Their purpose is not to represent official data collected scientifically, but rather to help the reader understand various mechanisms and processes. The value of the diagrams is qualitative rather than quantitative. Graphs are used to reinforce learning, not to demonstrate scientific evidence.

When we eat highly processed carbs such as baked goods, white flour, candy, or chips, and when we eat simple sugar such as the sugar in processed foods, baked goods, and sweet drinks, our blood sugar level rises quickly and high. To respond to that elevation of glucose in our bloodstream, our body releases insulin, a hormone that helps blood sugar (glucose) enter our cells for energy – brain cells included.

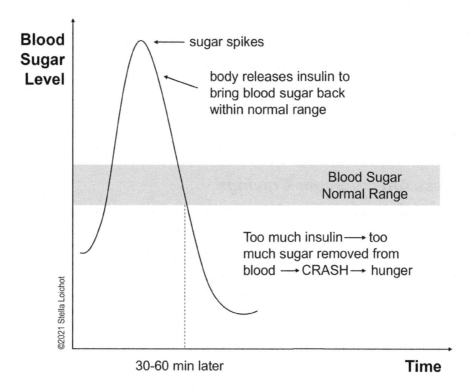

This process allows the sugar in our blood to go back to a reasonable level. People who don't produce enough insulin (type 1 diabetes) or people insensitive to insulin (type 2 diabetes) see glucose accumulate in their bloodstream because the glucose can't enter the cells and has nowhere else to go.

However, when there is a sudden rush of glucose in our blood, our body often overcompensates and releases too much insulin (unless one suffers from type 1 diabetes). As a result, too much sugar is removed from our bloodstream and absorbed by the cells, and our blood sugar level goes below the normal range. This makes us crash, feel sleepy, get irritable, and we reach for another source of quick energy.

Being Tired Makes Us Inactive

Though exercise doesn't always make us lose weight directly, being physically active supports our weight loss journey and helps replace body fat with leaner mass (muscle). The more muscle mass we carry, as opposed to body fat, the more calories we burn at rest, which is great for someone who is trying to lose weight or maintain their weight. In addition, exercise can improve overall physical health, mental health, and general well-being. This is where sleep deprivation can do a lot of damage. When you are exhausted, where do you find the energy to move your body? Tired people are not as physically active as well-rested people, and their weight loss journey is usually harder and bumpier without the support of physical activity.

Appetite Hormones Are No Match

It is now widely known that lack of sleep can lead to inefficient regulation of our metabolism and appetite. If we don't sleep enough, our hormones become out of balance. When we sleep only a few hours, our levels of ghrelin (the "hunger hormone") are high. As our sleep gets longer, the ghrelin goes down. At the same time, the exact opposite happens with leptin, a hormone that tells us we are full after we have eaten. Leptin is the "satiety hormone," or fullness hormone, if you will. The longer we sleep, the more leptin our body releases.

If we don't sleep enough (less than seven hours, as a rule of thumb), not only are we hungrier during the following day, but we also don't feel full after eating.[9] Improving the quality and amount of our sleep is the only way to win this hormone battle.

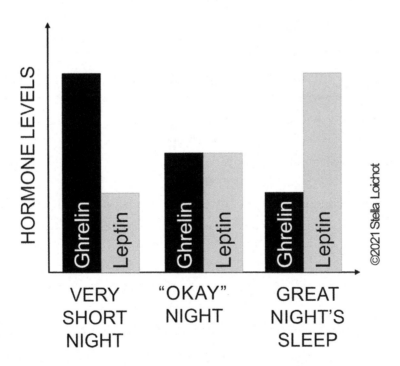

Less Sleep = More Fat, Less Muscle

Research has shown that people who are sleep-deprived while dieting lose muscle rather than fat.[10] If you plan to wake up an hour earlier every morning to go to the gym, but you have not added an extra hour of sleep into your evenings, you might want to rethink your strategy. The muscle mass you build during your morning workout might get lost just by not sleeping enough. Furthermore, as we will see later, deep sleep is linked to the production of growth hormones that enhance the utilization of fats by our muscles.[11]

If weight loss and weight management are on your radar, you don't want to dismiss this information. It is time to focus on your sleep, either its length or its quality.

For some people, it is tempting to rely solely on willpower, rather than proper sleep hygiene, to manage their weight. Yet, from experience, I know that relying on willpower for weight management is not a good idea. It is not sustainable in the long term and it often makes us miserable. I have found an easier and more reliable way to get results. Improving sleep quality and increasing sleep duration are part of the solution, even if sleep is the missing link that people seldom want to direct their attention to.

SLEEP AND TYPE 2 DIABETES

Type 2 diabetes, which is now the seventh leading cause of death in the United States, is a dangerous condition that can lead to heart disease, amputation, kidney failure, and blindness. Studies have shown that sleep deprivation can increase a person's chances of having type 2 diabetes.

Sleep deprivation causes two critical metabolic changes in the human body: a decrease in glucose tolerance and an increase in insulin resistance.[12]

Glucose intolerance and insulin resistance are syndromes predisposing to type 2 diabetes and the reason researchers "urge clinicians to recommend at least seven hours of uninterrupted sleep per night as part of a healthy lifestyle."[13]

How does it work?

When someone is chronically sleep-deprived, their body releases less insulin when they eat. As was mentioned before, insulin is the hormone that allows glucose (blood sugar) to enter our cells and provide them with energy. If there is not enough insulin released when we eat, glucose accumulates in our blood. Lack of sleep also leads to our body releasing more stress hormones, such as cortisol.[14] Cortisol, though it creates a sense of "awakeness," also makes insulin less effective. A sleep-deprived person releases less insulin, and this insulin is not as efficient. The consequences are huge: glucose accumulates in our blood and can damage our blood vessels, starting with the smallest ones. The parts of our body that have the smallest vessels (capillaries) usually suffer first from diabetes: our eyes, kidneys, and nervous system. Indeed, complications from type 2 diabetes include blindness, peripheral neuropathy, and permanent kidney damage.

Interestingly enough, these side effects have been observed not just for those who sleep very little but also for those who sleep six hours per night. Think about it: if we go to bed at 10 pm, read for a while, and then wake up twice during the night before getting up at 6 am the next day, chances are we will sleep about six hours each night. Sleeping six hours is not unusual for most people, and this less obvious lack of sleep negatively affects our ability to maintain proper insulin sensitivity and blood sugar management.[15]

When it comes to the ideal sleep duration, it seems that the lowest risk for type 2 diabetes is at seven to eight hours of sleep per day, according to a study looking at 482,502 participants for 2.5 to 16 years.[16]

Unfortunately, the link between lack of sleep and prediabetes or type 2 diabetes is often overlooked. When trying to reverse prediabetes or improve blood sugar levels, we tend to focus our efforts on weight loss, nutrition, and exercise, completely ignoring sleep. This is a colossal mistake, but one that can be corrected easily.

I regularly work with clients who have just been diagnosed with prediabetes. When they come to me, they explain that their doctor has recommended a healthier diet and more physical activity. These are great recommendations, but what I often witness is that my clients are too busy to incorporate healthy homemade meals and regular workouts in their lifestyle. Often, they cut into their sleep time to fit in these activities. Sleep is the only thing that they can reduce without apparent side effects, which they can hide with coffee, energy drinks, and sugary snacks. With this mindset, sleep becomes a luxury, and my clients become sleep-deprived.

To conquer type 2 diabetes, we have to consider sleep for what it is: a productive part of our life, not just wasted hours doing nothing.

SLEEP AND ATHLETIC PERFORMANCE

Being physically active has a significant impact on our weight but also on our ability to regulate blood sugar and thus avoid type 2 diabetes. It is recommended that an adult perform at least 150 to 300 minutes of moderate physical activity per week, or 75 to 150 minutes of intense physical activity per week, to reap health benefits.[17]

Unfortunately, increasing physical activity in our daily life is not an effortless task, and sleep deprivation can make it almost impossible to sustain.

We all know how it goes, though. We resolve to live a healthier life and hit the gym three or four times a week before heading off to work. We can do this, right? We are motivated! We want to be active, we want to be lean, and we want to build muscles. The alarm clock goes off at 4:30 am (two hours earlier than usual), and we jump into our gym clothes, feeling proud of our decision.

This plan could be a great one if every time we subtracted an hour of sleep in the morning, we went to bed an hour earlier the night before. Regrettably, we rarely do that.

Fortunately, most of us pay more and more attention to fitness and have realized over the past years that exercising makes a tremendous difference to wellness. Yet, according to Dr. Helene A. Emsellem, Medical Director of the Center for Sleep & Wake Disorders in Chevy Chase, Maryland, more and more people are trying to carve time out of their busy day to fit in a workout, and sleep often bears the consequences. "I see people sleep-deprived because they got up early to exercise," Dr. Emsellem says.[18]

Why is this a problem? It is commonly known that sleep deprivation affects memory, cognitive function, decision-making processes, etc. Yet we often assume — mistakenly — that we can compensate for lack of sleep by drinking an extra cup of coffee, eating an extra snack, or by making extra efforts to focus.

Lack of sleep also has an enormous impact on our body, our muscles, and, as a result, our athletic performance. Therefore, many people, despite training regularly and apparently "doing all the right things," struggle at improving their fitness level, their speed, their distances, and their strength. No one says it better than James B. Maas, Ph.D., Professor of Psychology at Cornell University. As the author of the book *Power Sleep* states, "Sleep is a necessity, not a luxury, especially for athletes."[19]

Have You Heard of hGH?

The release of human growth hormones (hGH) prompts cell growth and cell division and leads to tissue growth and repair. Though we release growth hormones during the day, there is a surge at night, especially shortly after the onset of sleep.[20] The release of growth hormones at night allows our muscles, tendons, and bones to repair, grow, and get stronger so we can be more powerful and less prone to injury during the day.

A study from Brunel University in the U.K. explains that sleep and exercise are the most powerful natural triggers of growth hormone secretion.[21]

It has been established that our body is programmed to release growth hormones during Slow Wave Sleep – also called deep sleep – and the release of these hormones is directly linked to the time we spend sleeping.

Growth hormones are mostly produced in the first few hours of the night. Their release is linked to our biological rhythm. This means that when our body is ready to release growth hormones, we need to be asleep for the release to happen properly.

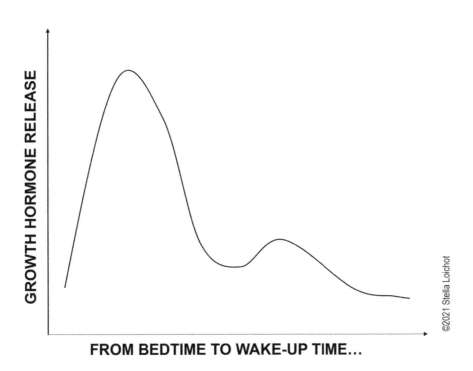

©2021 Stella Loichot

GROWTH HORMONE RELEASE

FROM BEDTIME TO WAKE-UP TIME...

If our body is programmed for us to sleep at 9 pm, growth hormones will mostly be released between about 9 pm and 12 am, as long as we are in a deep sleep at that time. But what happens if we go to bed at 11 pm? Our body misses out on about two hours of growth hormone release and will not be as strong the next day.

Of course, in actual life, this process is much more complex and variable, depending on the person, but looking at sleep this way gives us a better idea of what happens when we stay up later than we should. It also makes it clear why someone whose body needs to go to bed early and wake up early (an early bird) will miss out on hormone release if they regularly postpone their bedtime. A night owl who wakes up a bit too early every day might not suffer as much when it comes to growth hormone release but might experience other issues linked to sleep deprivation.

What Can Cheating Athletes Teach Us?

Growth hormones play an important role in sports performance[22] and are even used to artificially increase speed and endurance by some unscrupulous professional athletes.[23] One effect attributed to human growth hormones is "increased muscle mass and strength."[24] So, does it make sense to hit the gym every day if you are depriving yourself of the benefits of growth hormone release by sleeping less?

Working out is essential, but you might not get the expected results if your exercise routine comes at the expense of a good night's sleep. Getting up early? *Yes!* But then make sure you also go to bed earlier, to get a full and restful night, with all the deep sleep that your brain and body deserve. Going to bed late to fit in a workout at night so that you don't have to get up early the next day? Again, think twice. You might miss out on growth hormones, and exercising won't be as beneficial as it could be.

Recovery and Injury Prevention

When we are sleep-deprived and our body does not release enough growth hormones, our muscles cannot fully repair themselves after a workout. Not only does this lengthen your recovery time, but it also puts you at greater risk for injuries. Let's break down this process.

When we exercise, we are challenging the fibers that make up our muscles. This causes micro-tears, which often translate to soreness immediately after or a couple of days later. Those microscopic tears are normal, and they are part of the muscle growth process. When our body works to repair the "damaged" fibers, it builds an even stronger muscle, in anticipation of future stress during workouts. Therefore, regular exercise allows us to build stronger muscles.[25]

If we don't give muscles the time and nutrition to repair after each workout, they won't grow stronger and will even weaken because of the accumulation of micro-tears. This eventually leads to an increased risk of injury. Once again, if we forgo sleep for a longer workout, we are not doing ourselves a favor. Resting is as essential in an exercise routine as the workout itself.

The current diet and exercise trends urge you to always push further. Remember, you have the tools to stack all the odds in your favor and make sure your exercise routine does not take over your sleep routine. If your days are too packed to fit in both a workout and a good night's sleep, it is crucial that you try to find other activities to cut down on. Maybe spend less time on social media or in front of the TV. Spread out your grocery shopping trips. Or skip one or two meetings that are not critical. Making some room in your daily schedule could lead to a more fulfilling life.

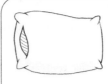

SPECIAL TIP

Sometimes, it is hard to decide what is our routine, and what is an exception. Here is a trick to help you define what YOU consider a "special situation." Imagine that you were working out once a month. Would you regard that as exceptional or a habit? Now imagine that you were working out twice a month? Would it be exceptional or a habit? What about once a week? Once you have decided on what is a habit and what is a special occasion for a workout, apply the same standards to your sleep. If you consider that going to the gym once a week is a habit, then don't assume that being sleep-deprived once a week is exceptional. We need to be aware of our tendency to have double standards, depending on what is convenient and brings us peace of mind.

For many of us, sleep is what we sacrifice when life becomes overwhelming and our schedules too full. Yet it is important, for us and for future generations, to accept the fact that sleep is not a malleable part of the day that we can stretch or compress on a whim. Once we know how much sleep we need to function optimally (or at least well!), we need to commit to it and keep it as regular as possible. Sometimes, life gets in the way, and we don't sleep as much as we need to for a few nights. That is fine, as long as it is only occasionally.

Fat Metabolism

Not only are growth hormones important for fitness, but they also help our body use more fat for energy by enhancing our ability to break down triglycerides.[26]

It is essential to optimize our body's utilization of fat for several reasons. For example, our fat storage, however lean we are, can keep us going for hours and hours, which is especially important for endurance. Furthermore, increasing fat metabolism is just another way to say "burning fat," which is one of the principal reasons many of us work out in the first place.

Beyond exercise, it is important to keep in mind that tapping into our fat reserves (triglycerides) also helps reduce their concentration in the bloodstream, which lowers the risk of heart disease associated with high concentrations of triglycerides in the blood.[27] Too much fat in our body is also a risk factor for insulin resistance and type 2 diabetes.

Improved Immune System

Sleep helps boost our immune system and allows us to fight diseases, colds, infections, and more.[28] Because illnesses can completely derail a training plan, having a strong immune system and being able to prioritize sleep is extremely important when it comes to showing up to the gym, feeling good on race day, or making it to each practice.

Increased Mental Focus and Strength

Sleep also plays a huge role in memory building, learning, decision making, and helping us be more focused. These functions are important for athletic performance and following a training plan.

Athletic performance might not be a priority for most of us. Still, sleep can help us move in our everyday lives with a lower risk of injury. This is especially important as we grow older and our ability to recover from physical damage starts declining.

MORE POWER TO SLEEP

The effects of sleep deprivation go way beyond impeding weight loss, furthering diabetes, and decreasing fitness. It is essential to know about the dangers of lack of sleep to develop the profound motivation required to change our habits. Knowing the facts might be what enables us to work on our sleep habits for months and find success, rather than trying a few strategies and giving up.

Stroke

A study conducted by the University of Alabama, which observed 5,666 adults over three years, showed that middle- to older-aged people of normal weight, who regularly got fewer than six hours of sleep per night, were four times more likely to have strokes, even if they didn't have a history of stroke, than normal-weight people who were getting seven to eight hours of sleep.[29]

Heart Attack

Leading academics from the University of War-wick Medical School in the UK discovered that an adult who regularly sleeps less than five or six hours per night and experiences poor quality sleep might have a 48% greater chance of developing or dying from coronary heart disease.[30]

Alzheimer's Disease

It has long been known that people with Alzheimer's disease, besides losing their memory, often struggle with sleep. What has also been discovered recently is that it also works the other way

DID YOU KNOW?
Research has shown that the neurons in our brain shrink while we are deeply asleep. This process is vital because it gives our lymphatic system room to clean out any toxins that have accumulated between them.[32]

If our brain can't clean itself up as it should, we might have an elevated risk of developing dementia and Alzheimer's disease.[33]

around. According to research funded by the National Institutes of Health (NIH), chronic lack of sleep can lead to an accumulation of toxic protein in the brain that worsens memory loss and speeds up the disease's progression and the cognitive decline that comes with Alzheimer's.[31]

Many processes happen in our body and brain while we sleep, which we will not review in detail here. We regenerate our cells and get rid of the toxins and free radicals that make us age faster and put us at risk for inflammation and disease. According to research from the University of Warwick, short sleepers see a 12% increase in their risk of dying prematurely compared to those who usually sleep six to eight hours each night.[34]

· · ·

So, is there no hope?

If you are not sleeping well, sustainable weight loss might be impossible, and avoiding type 2 diabetes or another chronic disease will most likely feel like an uphill battle, if not a lost cause. It does not mean that you are doomed or will inevitably face all these consequences later on. Being motivated to change is the first step. Going forward, things can only get better.

Obviously, it is important to work on improving your sleep as soon as you can. But it matters less whether you get it "fixed" in two weeks, two months, or one year. What counts is that you work on your sleep right away and gradually restore it.

It is essential to take one step at a time without the pressure to succeed. As stated by Dr. Patrick Lemoine, psychiatrist and director of clinical training at Claude Bernard University in Lyon, France, the number one obstacle to falling asleep is actually the pressure to fall asleep. In a radio show aired in January 2019, Dr. Lemoine described the following experiment that was done with 30 adults who had no issues with sleep at all and had never experienced insomnia. They gathered all the subjects in a dormitory where they had to spend the night. Just before turning the light off for the night, they promised the subjects 10,000 euros to the first person who would fall asleep. None of them could sleep that night. They all stayed awake, as the desire to sleep and the stakes were so high that it made drifting into sleep impossible.[35]

It might take you a month to improve your sleep, or it might take you a year. The strategies and tools presented in this book should help you tremendously, whether you do it alone or with a coach, a doctor, or a therapist. Bottom line: just get started!

CHAPTER TWO
How Sleep-Deprived Are You?

Until the day I collapsed, I had no clue I was sleep-deprived. In hindsight, it is beyond understanding that I didn't see what was going on, but at the time, it didn't occur to me that I was actually on my last legs. Don't get me wrong: I felt drained and fatigued emotionally and physically, but I blamed it on my career, on my triathlon training, on my responsibilities as a mother. I blamed my exhaustion on all the things I was doing, rather than acknowledging what I was NOT doing: sleeping. Why didn't I connect the dots? Honestly, I am still not sure. Maybe because I didn't want to know. Or because I felt worn out but not sleepy per se. Maybe sleep had so little value in my eyes that I didn't even think of it. It was most likely a combination of all these reasons. But the chief reason was that I had built an entire system of coping mechanisms. Because I knew that a minor glitch in my "perfect life" would have knocked me to the ground, my stress level was sky-high, and my body was flooded with cortisol (which was confirmed by blood work a little later). At the same time, I was pumped full of endorphins from daily workouts, the adrenaline from the races, and a pot of coffee every day. I didn't get a chance to feel sleepy during the day unless I took a break and relaxed, which I happily avoided since it felt uncomfortable and did nothing but get me behind in my goals.

One day, I fell asleep in the YMCA hot tub. A lady woke me up as my head started falling into the water. When I talked to the doctors, they told me to take naps, but I saw no way to fit them into my schedule. I knew they were right but didn't want to listen because it made me feel helpless. I could feel something was wrong but didn't know how and what to change, so my only choice seemed to be to keep pushing forward, in search of even more adrenaline to make up for the lack of sleep. I don't think anyone was aware that I was sleep-deprived. I honestly wasn't. I loved my life. The action was intoxicating, and even though I could feel the sword of Damocles above my head, I didn't see the need to change my ways and make room for sleep, as long as I could keep it all together.

Where did the wake-up call come from? It was brutal. I became ill, and from one day to the next, I had to stop exercising: no more running, biking, or swimming. That's when my body collapsed. Suddenly, I had no way to maintain a high level of endorphins, dopamine, or adrenaline. My sources of energy were gone. I also ended up with 13 hours of free time every week because that is how much I had been working out before. With all that free time on my hands, my level of stress went down drastically, and it pushed me out of fight-or-flight mode for the first time in years. I had nothing to keep me going, and pots of caffeine couldn't do anything to pick me up. I was a mess.

Even walking became a challenge. I remember hitting rock bottom one day, walking back from school with my three daughters. It was only half a mile, but I couldn't do it. I took a break, sitting on the sidewalk, wondering how I could find the strength to make it home. A teacher from my kids' school was driving by and gave us all a ride. Sitting in his dark green station wagon was when it hit me: I had to change; I had to sleep. Not just because I was sick at that time but for decades to come. I came home and cried. Life as I knew it was over.

This might sound ridiculous, and maybe you wonder how someone could be that foolish to dismiss sleep entirely and get to that point of distress. I am not an exception, and as a Health and Behavioral Change Coach, I work every single day with clients who are sleep-deprived without realizing it, which is the very first step to making lifestyle changes.

How could I be so oblivious?

As members of society, we usually identify our needs and gauge whether or not they are met by comparing our circumstances to those of others in our community. Whether it is sleep or financial resources, most of us end up being comfortable with what's considered the "norm." If you live in an old trailer parked on the street of an upper-class neighborhood where residents keep their brand-new trailer in three-car garages next to their yacht, you will likely feel poor. If you take that same trailer and park it next to a homeless encampment, chances are you will feel privileged and lucky.

It is the same with sleep. If you sleep seven hours each night but your family and friends go to bed later than you and wake up earlier, you might assume that you sleep enough. You might even feel slightly lazy and guilty when your colleague tells you all about her daily 4:30 am fitness boot camp. Even if you are tired, you won't assume that you are sleep-deprived; you will just blame it on hormones, stress, or some kind of mysterious health issue. You might be right, by the way! On the other hand, if everyone around you sleeps nine hours per night and you are stuck at seven hours, you will either believe that you are a blessed alien if you don't feel tired or will realize that you are not getting enough snooze and will be more inclined to try to make some changes.

The problem is, we live in a society where lack of sleep is widespread and goes unnoticed most of the time.

Though sleep is instrumental in the development of good health and mental or physical performance, many people are trying to cut back on sleep. Sleeping less is the recent trend in our fast-paced Western society. More and more people are commuting or working out at 4 am, and somehow, they are still bringing work home and sending work emails at 11 pm.

When she was Associate Director of Sleep Disorders at the Boston Medical Center, Yelena Pyatkevich explained that we, as a society, have lost one hour and a half of sleep each night over the past 100 years.[1] This would amount to one month and a half of sleep per year, or ten years by the time we reach 80 years old. The World Health Organization confirms that globally, nightly sleep time has been reduced by 20% over the past century.[2]

 DID YOU KNOW?
Studies show that 67% of French people wake up after 7 am,[5] while more than half of Americans are up by 6:30 am.[6] For Spanish women, the average wake up time is actually after 8 am (Kluger 2016).[7] Why is this important to mention? Because it reminds us that our habits are rooted in our culture and policies. The way we do things is not necessarily the way we *have* to do things and definitely not the "right" way to do things. If schooling, work, or your commute requires you to get up early even though you are not an early bird, it doesn't mean that there is something wrong with you. There is no right or wrong, there is just you, what you need, and what you can do. Of course, you still need to figure out a way to make things work, but don't assume that *you* need to be fixed. In another country, maybe your natural sleep patterns would fit perfectly with everybody else's.

Almost a third of Americans sleep less than six hours,[3] and this tendency, called "short sleep" (less than six hours), has become an increasing trend since 2013.[4] Fortunately, we can reverse the trend by making a conscious effort to sleep more.

Here is what is sure: sleep in our society has lost its perceived value. We have come to a point where sleeping less is something to show off. How many times have you heard someone brag about sleeping only five hours per night? Or about the fact that they get up five times a week at 4 am to go work out? We seem to find pride in not sleeping well or not sleeping enough. We have to change this entire culture of sleep deprivation. It starts with *your* feeling proud about taking care of your sleep rather than feeling guilty for wanting to sleep more.

I am not implying that the time we get up in the morning or the time we go to bed at night is based solely on our actions and decisions. There is no level playing field, and some of us struggle with insanely long commutes, taxing jobs, and other demands from life that interfere with a good night's sleep. In my work, though, I often see clients who are, by pure choice, responsible for their lack of sleep but don't realize it because they don't have the time to sit back and reflect on their life and daily habits. Being aware and determined to sleep better is the very first step in this journey.

Being sleep-deprived doesn't always mean feeling exhausted. Most of us function just fine without enough sleep. Unfortunately, there is an enormous difference between functioning "just fine" and functioning optimally. Our sleep deprivation can go unnoticed in the same way that we get used to a mild chronic pain until it worsens or disappears. Not only are we not aware of sleep deprivation, but we often unconsciously compensate for it (using coffee, soda, exercise, etc.). Though we do not notice it, our body and our brain are not functioning at their maximum capacity.

WHAT'S YOUR SLEEP SCORE?

Below are three easy ways for you to assess whether you might be sleep-deprived. Taking these tests cannot be used in place of any form of diagnosis, and it is important that you seek help from a qualified healthcare professional if you are struggling with your sleep. Feeling sleepy during the day is not just linked to sleep deprivation. It can also come from erratic blood sugar levels, vitamin deficiency, poor digestion, etc. Consider these tests as self-awareness tools and keep in mind that if you do feel sleep-deprived, you probably are, regardless of what the tests may show.

Sleep Quiz

On the following page is a short quiz that helps you find out whether or not you sleep enough. I use this quiz in my practice. It is based on personal exploration and on what I have observed with the adults I work with. It is a good starting point based on anecdotal experience. It is mostly inspired by the Epworth Sleepiness Scale created by John Murray Jones and based on scientific research.[8] I don't find the Epworth Sleepiness Scale very easy to apply to real-life situations – which is why I developed my own quiz – but you might appreciate the fact that it is backed up by science.

To find out how sleep-deprived you might be, check the appropriate column next to each real-life situation. All the checkmarks in column #1 are worth one point, checkmarks in column #2 are

Sleep Quiz

Available online

1. Check the most appropriate response to each situation.
2. Multiply check marks in each column by the point value for that column.
3. Add up the points to find out your Sleep Score.
The higher the score, the better!

For a full report and personalized tips, take this quiz online!

Could this happen to you?	Yes (1 pt)	Maybe (2 pts)	No (3 pts)
Fall asleep when resting or reading during the day			
Wake up tired and not recharged			
Easily fall asleep as a passenger in a car			
Grab a snack during the day to fight off sleepiness			
Plan a 10-minute nap and wake up 1 hour later			
Doze off during a play, movie, or concert			
Snooze during a meeting			
Drink more than 2 caffeinated beverages per day			
Sleep at least 2 hours longer on weekends			
Fall asleep, without intending to, while watching TV			
Points Per Column			
YOUR SLEEP SCORE			

worth two points, and checkmarks in column #3 are worth three points. Once you have added all the points, you get a total score between 10 and 30. The lower your score, the more you need to work on your sleep.

For an easier way to take this quiz, and if you would like to receive customized tips to help you change your sleeping habits, check out the online version of this quiz at allonZcoaching.com/sleepitoff. Your results will be compiled automatically, and you'll receive a personalized email with suggestions on how to improve your sleep.

Spoon Test

The spoon test, which is also called the Sleep Onset Latency Test, can help you determine the severity of your sleep deprivation. It is a fun complement to the Sleep Quiz or Epworth Sleepiness Scale. The spoon test was created by Dr. Nathaniel Kleitman from the University of Chicago, who is known as the "father of sleep research" and lived to 104 years old![9]

To run this test, all you need is a watch, a metal spoon, and a metal tray. Note that this test is not meant to be done at night!

First, lie down on the edge of a bed or couch in a dark room. You need to be comfortable enough to fall asleep, so pick the position that feels right to you. Set a large metal tray beside the bed and hold your spoon in your hand, right over the tray. Record the time and close your eyes with the intent of falling asleep.

If you fall asleep, you let go of the spoon and are awakened by the noise of it hitting the tray. Record the time right away. If it has been less than 15 minutes, you are probably not sleeping enough. If it took you longer than 15 minutes to fall asleep or if you didn't fall asleep at all, there is a chance that you are not sleep-deprived.

A more convenient way to run this test is to set a timer for 15 minutes and see whether you fall asleep within that time frame.

Though this test is worth trying, it might not work for everyone since some people, although very sleep-deprived, find it hard to fall asleep during the day because their brain is too alert. They find it hard to "let go."

Coffee Test

If you are a coffee drinker, here is a super simple test that you can do: quit coffee for ten days and see how it goes! If you find that you're dragging yourself along all day, battling between a headache and a lack of energy, it means you are not sleeping enough. Caffeine has been masking your sleep deprivation, and it is time to change your habits. To reduce withdrawal symptoms and limit risks of falling asleep when you don't want to, you can cut back gradually.

Sometimes, the headache and apathy caused by caffeine withdrawal may fade after a few days, and you may start feeling good again. If this is the case for you, try to cut back on coffee in your daily routine. You can either drink less every day or drink it less regularly to keep your body from developing an addiction. Drinking coffee regularly can only impair your sleeping habits, so it is an excellent idea to limit it as much as possible.

Regarding the results you get in these tests, remember that you know your body best. If you feel sleep-deprived but get contradictory results, it is important to trust yourself and know that you need more sleep or better-quality sleep.

CAREFULLY ASSESS YOUR SLEEP

There are two distinct causes of sleep deprivation: not sleeping enough is one. Not sleeping well is the other. Some people combine them: they don't sleep enough, and when they sleep, it is not a sound and refreshing sleep. Both aspects, duration and quality of sleep, are equally important. We will come back to sleep quality later, but for now, it is critical to assess how many hours of sleep you get regularly.

How Many Hours Do You Dedicate to Sleep?

It is easy to know how much time we spend in bed, but a little trickier to find out how many hours we spend asleep. There is a difference between lying in bed reading, checking the news, watching TV, shopping online, or cuddling with our partner and actually being asleep. To get an accurate idea of the time you dedicate to sleep, track your sleep for at least one week.

The Sleep Tracker is meant to gather more data than just the hours you dedicate to sleep. Record as much information as possible for at least one week, rather than spending a week tracking only the hours you devote to sleep and then spending another week or two tracking other parameters of your sleep. See the example on the next page. If you track everything at once, you will gather a ton of valuable information about your sleep that we will use later.

Sleep Tracker 1/2

	1	2	3	4	5
	Turn off lights & try to sleep at:	Fall asleep at:	Awake during the night	Next day wake-up time	Stop trying to fall back to sleep at:
Friday	midnight	midnight	15 min	9:15 am	9:15 am
Saturday	1:30 am	around 2 am	0	5:15 am	10:00 am
Sunday	11:45 pm	midnight	30 min	7:00 am	7:00 am
Monday	11 pm	Around 11 pm	0	7:00 am	7:00 am
...					

Sleep Tracker 1/2

Download online

Track your sleep for at least a full week.

	1	2	3	4	5
	Turn off lights & try to sleep at:	Fall asleep at:	Awake during the night	Next day wake-up time	Stop trying to fall back to sleep at:
Friday					
Saturday					
Sunday					
Monday					
Tuesday					
Wednesday					
Thursday					

On the next page, report the following calculations:

Time Dedicated to Sleep = Time elapsed between column #1 and column #5

Time Actually Asleep = Time elapsed between column #2 and column #4, minus column #3

You don't have to be super accurate, you are just trying to get a better idea of what is going on.

33

Following the example on page 32, start tracking your sleep using the Sleep Tracker provided in the ready-to-print workbook that is available for download at allonZcoaching.com/sleepitoff. You will need to use the password SLEEP_IT_OFF to access the workbook.

By the time you have filled out all the columns of the Sleep Tracker for at least a week, you have accumulated a lot of useful data that can help you improve your sleep with this step-by-step guide. Generally, I don't recommend keeping such a close eye on the clock when in bed. Checking the time might create stress due to the fear of being tired the next day, and it can be a significant source of anxiety. Furthermore, checking the time when we wake up in the middle of the night puts us in a state of alertness that is not desirable for falling back to sleep. But to evaluate your current sleep, it is necessary to monitor the clock. For most people, tracking for one week or two is enough to get excellent-quality information.

To find out how many hours you devote to sleep each night, focus on columns #1 and #5. Look at the times recorded in those two columns and find out how many hours have gone by between the time you started trying to sleep (and doing nothing else) and the time you stopped trying to fall back asleep the next morning. If you wake up during the night (column #3) and do nothing more than try to go back to sleep, the time you spend lying awake counts as time that you are dedicating to sleep, so don't even pay attention to that column for now. On the other hand, if you get up to let the dog out, check on the kids, or read your emails, you need to deduct the time you spend doing these activities from the total hours you dedicate to sleep.

Calculating how many hours you sleep can be annoying. If you don't want to do it yourself, you can use an online time calculator for assistance. Visit allonZcoaching.com/sleepitoff for a link to a user-friendly time calculator.

When we track our sleep, we must be honest. We are not trying to judge ourselves. The goal of this tracker is to get an accurate snapshot of our nighttime sleep so that we can identify any problems and fix them. Report your results in the worksheet on page 36.

If, after analyzing the data in your Sleep Tracker, you realize that you are not allocating enough time to sleep every night, you know what to work on. Though more work needs to be done, this is still a great starting point.

Sleep Tracker 2/2

Example

	Time Dedicated to Sleep	Time Actually Asleep
Friday	9h 15min	9h
Saturday	8h 30min	3h 15min
Sunday	7h 15min	6h 30min
Monday	8h	8h

What do you notice when looking at your results?

I sleep way less than I thought. Schedule is irregular

What can you change? Where can you improve?

Spend less time on phone in bed and sleep instead.

Plan bedtime according to wake-up time to have

at least 8.5 hours

Sleep Tracker 2/2

Download online

Report your Sleep Results Below.

	Time Dedicated to Sleep	Time Actually Asleep
Friday		
Saturday		
Sunday		
Monday		
Tuesday		
Wednesday		
Thursday		

What do you notice when looking at your results?

_____

_____

What can you change? Where can you improve?

_____

_____

You need to plan enough time in your established routine for regeneration, recovery, and learning, or you might compromise your health and energy. Dedicating over a third of your life to "doing nothing" might be a challenge. Still, it is crucial for you to start thinking about how you can prioritize sleep and aim for about eight hours of actual sleep.

How Many Hours Do You Actually Sleep?

There is often a discrepancy between the time we think we allocate to sleep and the real sleep time we are getting. Many of us spend a lot of time in bed, yet not sleeping at all. Not only because we do other things while in bed, but also because it takes time to fall asleep. The mistake most of us make is that if we plan on sleeping eight hours, we go to bed eight hours before our alarm clock goes off the next morning.

By filling out this Sleep Tracker, you can see clearly that the time that goes by between Column #1 and Column #2 cannot be neglected. If we go to bed at 10 pm and have to wake up at 6 am, there is no way we can sleep for eight hours. If you calculate the time elapsed between column #1 and column #5, you get the time you dedicate to sleep. For most people, this time has not much to do with actual sleep time.

Estimating how long we sleep can be tricky because we don't know exactly when we fall asleep (column #2 of the Sleep Tracker). Electronic tracking devices (watch, phone app, etc.) can help somewhat in that regard, even if they don't all deliver the same accuracy. If you want to use an electronic device to record your sleep temporarily, make sure you do your research and find a device that does more than just monitor your visible body movement throughout the night. You might want to look into devices monitoring also your heart rate and your breathing.

When and How Long Should You Track?

Monitor your sleep for one or two weeks. Tracking your sleep for a brief period gives you awareness of your habits. It might also help you understand what is going on during the night that is keeping you from sleeping well.

Keep in mind that tracking your sleep for longer than a few weeks can be detrimental to your sleep for two reasons.

First, tracking your sleep might keep you from relaxing before bed because it maintains your brain in a state of alertness and keeps you awake. Disconnecting from everything is necessary for a good night's sleep. We will talk more about that later. Technology keeps us alert, which means that it activates our sympathetic nervous system. This is the system that is turned on when we are stressed (whether it is good stress or bad stress), and this is the system that needs to be shut down for us to fall and stay asleep.

The second reason is that when you focus too hard on your sleep, whether with a tracking device or with a paper log, it can easily turn into an obsession that causes a lot of anxiety. Worrying about insomnia is sometimes enough to create and perpetuate insomnia. If you go to bed at night worried that you might not sleep well, chances are you will have difficulty falling and staying asleep. To sleep properly, we need to let go of any worries or thoughts, and tracking our sleep for too long could make this very difficult.

Once you have collected the data you need to improve your sleep, keep your phone and other devices out of the bedroom (or at least turned off). This is one of the first and most important actions you can take to optimize your nights.

SLEEP-DEPRIVED: NOW WHAT?

Acknowledging that you don't sleep enough, or not well enough, is the only way you can start making lifestyle changes. Maybe you are not as foolish as I was and you already know that you are sleep-deprived. If that's the case, that's great, but don't assume that testing your sleep with the tools provided in this chapter is pointless. The data you compile by tracking your sleep will help you know where you are starting from and give you a benchmark to evaluate your progress as you make changes in your life. The data will also give you a better idea of what to aim for, which is critical if you want to succeed.

This newly gained knowledge is not enough, though. Just as knowing that sleep is critical to your cognitive functions or that the amount of sleep you get heavily impacts your weight and blood sugar won't make you sleep better, knowing that you are sleep-deprived won't make you sleep more. It is now time to move to the next step and understand how sleep actually works.

CHAPTER THREE
The Mechanics Of Sleep

"I know what I should do, but I don't do it! Not sure why . . ."

You cannot even imagine how often I hear that in my practice. We usually know what we "should" do. That doesn't mean that we do it or that we can do it. The chief reason is that we often need support and guidance. Hopefully, this book will provide some of that. The second reason is that we don't quite understand how things work. As a result, we have a broad idea of what we "should" do but are not confident about what it means exactly and how it can be applied to our specific circumstances. We don't know where to start, so we don't start at all. Imagine a car mechanic who doesn't know how an engine runs. They would be clueless about how to fix your stalling vehicle.

The same applies to sleep, and if you are serious about improving the quality of your sleep, it is now time to learn more about the basic machinery of sleep so you feel confident enough to make changes that will bring you results.

SLEEP CYCLE AND BRAIN WAVES

Our brain cells continuously communicate with each other via electric waves. When we are awake, these waves move quickly. This puts us in a state of alertness that allows our body to function correctly, and we can think, act, fight, or run away if needed. When we sleep, these brain waves slow down. The speed of the brain waves depends on where we are in our sleep cycle. Throughout a typical night, we go through several sleep cycles. During each sleep cycle, we move through different stages of sleep, going from light sleep to deep sleep and rapid eye movement (REM) sleep, and then back to lighter sleep for the start of a new cycle.[1] When we have trouble falling asleep at night or when we wake up in the middle of the night and can't go back to sleep, it is often because our brain waves are too fast and their length is too close to what it is during the day.

Each sleep cycle looks a little like the chart below. The different length of each stage is not represented here because the duration of each stage varies greatly depending on the person, their age, and also whether they are going through that specific cycle at the beginning or the end of the night.

Stage one is an introduction to sleep. Brain waves start slowing down so we can enter stage two, a transition phase that allows us to get into a deeper sleep.

DID YOU KNOW?
When we are sleep-deprived, our body gives priority to deep sleep, the stages that allow us to recover and regenerate, to the detriment of REM sleep. This is one reason why, even when we are sleep-deprived, we sometimes feel fine and can go for weeks or months of deprivation without noticing the effect on our health.

For our brain to change frequency from fast waves (awake) to slower waves (asleep), we need to relax and calm down. For some people, it is easy. For others, and during specific periods of life that are especially stressful, it is much more difficult. In such situations, we need to consciously help our system slow down, by using relaxation techniques such as meditation or cardiac coherence techniques, for example, but also by crafting a lifestyle and a sleep environment that will allow our mind to "slow down" and keep it from picking up cues of external threats. All through this book, we will review many techniques that can help in this regard.

Stages in a Typical Sleep Cycle

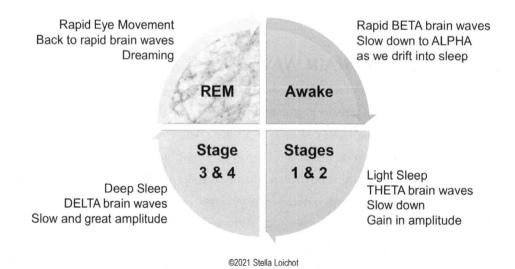

Rapid Eye Movement
Back to rapid brain waves
Dreaming

REM

Rapid BETA brain waves
Slow down to ALPHA
as we drift into sleep

Awake

Stage 3 & 4

Stages 1 & 2

Deep Sleep
DELTA brain waves
Slow and great amplitude

Light Sleep
THETA brain waves
Slow down
Gain in amplitude

©2021 Stella Loichot

It is when we are in stages three and four that our brain waves are the slowest. This is the deep-sleep phase of our sleep cycle. In those two stages, we recover, regenerate, and rest our bodies. We spend more time in a deep sleep during the first hours of the night, which makes those hours critical for good health. If our brain waves don't reach the slow frequency of deep sleep, or if our deep sleep is interrupted by faster waves, we wake up feeling tired, no matter how long we slept, because we don't get a chance to recharge. Younger people spend more time in stages three and four than older people do: about two hours per night for someone under 30 and about 30 minutes for someone over 65.[2]

DID YOU KNOW?
The name Rapid Eye Movement sleep is not an accurate description. People born without eyes can still dream and enjoy the benefits of REM sleep.

After deep sleep, we transition to what is called rapid eye movement sleep. REM is a phase in our sleep cycle during which our brain waves become faster than in deep sleep. During this time, our brain actively sorts through and stores information gathered during the day. REM sleep is when the brain does all the learning based on what we experienced the previous day. REM is a critical phase, especially in children, who have a longer REM cycle than adults. REM sleep is also when we dream. Because of this, our brain is quite active in this stage, but it still shouldn't be as active as during the day. If our brain waves are as fast as they are during the day, we wake up. We spend more time in REM sleep as the night progresses. This is one reason why, if we wake up naturally in the morning, chances are we'll wake up from a dream.

Knowing about the four stages of sleep gives us an informed perspective on our sleep patterns and sleep issues because it helps us understand that an external trigger (such as a blinking light or a distant noise) or an internal trigger (such as the need to use the restroom or poor digestion) will affect our sleep differently, depending on the stage we are in when it happens.

DID YOU KNOW?
In REM sleep, brain activity is very high. Yet certain parts of the brain are not activated, such as the area responsible for logic and structure. Therefore, our dreams are often very incoherent and overly emotional.

BIOLOGICAL CLOCK AND CHRONOTYPE

Our biological clock is an internal "clock" that dictates the timing of natural behaviors and bodily functions, such as sleeping, eating, and rises and falls in our blood pressure or body temperature.

According to a study by Czeisler et al. at Harvard University, the biological clock of healthy adults goes through an entire circadian cycle in about 24 hours and 11 minutes.[3] Put simply, it means that if we were to be in a room devoid of all light with no idea of the time of day, our body would adjust to a natural schedule where a full day would last, on average, 24 hours and 11 minutes rather than 24 hours.[4]

If we were not subject to external factors such as daylight disappearing at night and reappearing in the morning, we would tend to go to bed a bit later every day (by about 11 minutes).

For those of us who tend to push back our bedtime, know that this is partly physiological. These 24 hours and 11 minutes are an average, so some of us have a circadian cycle that's a bit longer or shorter. For the people who have a longer cycle, the temptation to go to bed later day after day can be strong. The risk of sleep deprivation becomes even higher if they still want to live according to a typical day/night schedule.

Our biological clock determines when we get sleepy and when we are naturally ready to wake up, independently of how tired we are or what we have done that day. In other words, our internal biological clock determines what we call our chronotype or, in more common terms, whether we are a night owl or an early bird.

Depending on their chronotype, some people are awake and productive late at night. In contrast, others reach their peak performance early in the morning.

Most people are neither evening nor morning people. They are a bit of both and quite flexible and adaptable: their biological clock adjusts very

 DID YOU KNOW?
Have you heard of French speleologist Michel Siffre? He spent two months in a cave in southern France with no cue from outside regarding the time of day (whether it was dark or bright). He had to estimate for himself when it was time to wake up, eat, or go to sleep. He had to keep track of time entirely on his own: no watch, no news. When he got out of the cave, after two months of isolation, he thought he had spent way less time in the cave than he actually had, because his biological clock had settled on a slightly longer circadian cycle than 24 hours.[5]

well to the environment and life's requirements. These people can usually thrive on pretty much any schedule that allows them to sleep around eight hours per night.

Only a tiny portion of the adult population has a chronotype that allows them to be highly productive both at night and early in the morning. These people need much less sleep than the average and are happy going to bed late and still waking up early. They sleep very little yet feel great and function at top levels without crutches such as coffee and energy drinks. According to many sleep experts, this is the case for only about 3 to 6% of adults. It might be tempting to assume we are one of these lucky people, but remember, compensating for tiredness with food and drink can keep us from noticing our sleep

 DID YOU KNOW?
Experiencing jet lag is very similar to adjusting to a schedule that doesn't fit your chronotype. Jet lag from traveling to the East is often harder to adjust to than jet lag from traveling to the West. Why? Because it is easier for us to stay awake when our biological clock tells us it is time to sleep than it is to fall asleep when our clock tells us we should be awake. And because it is easier to delay our bedtime, it is often what happens in real life: early birds tend to adjust to the night owls around them. It is not always the best option though, since early birds will miss out on deep sleep when they go to bed later than their body requires.

deprivation. High levels of stress, a lot of caffeine, or regular workouts throughout the day can help us ease the apparent symptoms of sleep deprivation. Unfortunately, these quick fixes won't keep us from developing chronic issues such as a weakened immune system, poor decision making, obesity, type 2 diabetes, or Alzheimer's. When we are trying to evaluate our sleep, it is essential to be honest with ourselves and acknowledge the external energy booster we rely on to make it through our day.

Our biological clocks make us spend more time in deep sleep in the first hours of the night and more time in lighter sleep as the night goes on. If you are neither an early bird nor a night owl, as is my case, luckily, your biological clock can adjust pretty quickly to reasonable variations in your sleep schedule. This means that if you go to bed a bit earlier or later than usual, you can still fully benefit from deep sleep and won't feel much of an impact on your body, as long as you sleep long enough.

But what happens if an early bird is trying to adjust to their night-owl spouse and goes to bed two or three hours "too late" every night compared to what their body needs? They could end up sleep-deprived very quickly, and it could easily lead to depression and other health issues. Why? Because they miss out on the first three hours of their biological night, the most restorative part of the night. That's also when growth hormones are released that help our bodies regenerate and repair. If we skip those three hours because we are not going to bed early enough, we are missing out on the most regenerative aspect of deep sleep.

It is often healthier for a night owl to slightly adjust their schedule and lifestyle to go to bed a little earlier. They might find it hard to fall asleep at first, but with good practice and rituals, they may slowly adjust. The key aspect here is that by going to bed earlier, they don't miss out on deep sleep, whereas early birds do when they postpone their bedtime.[6] Of course, night owls don't want to ignore their chronotype either, but adopting a slightly earlier bedtime won't have as significant an impact as it would for a morning person going to bed too late.

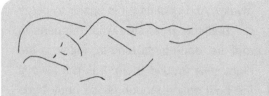

STORYTIME

When Josh started working with me, he was convinced that if he could sleep whenever he wanted, he would never fall asleep before 3 am and would sleep every single day until about 1 pm. This is actually the sleeping schedule he would implement when he was on vacation, and he felt good with that pattern as long as he could sleep in in the morning. Obviously, it was not realistic to keep such sleeping habits with a 9 to 5 job. Josh was exhausted and his mind felt foggy. He had to rely on caffeine and had a hard time finding the energy for regular workouts. He was also frustrated that he could not lose the few extra pounds he had gained over the past five years around his mid-section. Frustration and fatigue were impacting his relationship with his fiancée. He was becoming increasingly snappy with her and his sex drive was low, which made him very unhappy and insecure.

It didn't take long to get Josh back to a "normal" schedule. He is definitely a night owl, but his lifestyle had dramatically amplified his natural pattern. With a few intentional steps, he went back to a schedule that could accommodate both his biological clock and the demands of his career. The very first step (and the hardest one!) was for Josh to give up coffee for a few weeks while establishing a routine of always getting up and going to bed at the same time. After a month, he included intense physical activity early in the day and added a short night stroll to his bedtime routine. One thing that became clear after a few weeks of our working together was that Josh was eating too much during the second part of the day, and this was leading to acid reflux that kept him from feeling comfortable enough to fully relax and fall asleep at a reasonable time. Once he distributed his meals differently over the course of a day, he could fall asleep much earlier. He is now usually asleep by 11:30 pm and wakes up at 8 am every day, if not naturally, at least rested and recharged, ready for a day of productive work. The scale has tipped in the right direction, and Josh is finally on his way to reaching his goals after several years of stalling.

Research has shown that there are about two to three hours of difference, biologically, between early birds and night owls. That means that a night owl's body wants to go to bed only about two or three hours later than the body of a morning person.[7] What often happens, though, is that each of us tends to amplify our chronotype. Night owls tend to go to bed even later than their chronotype requires. Early birds often set their alarm clock even earlier than the time at which they would wake up naturally. It can lead some people to extreme sleep patterns and a feeling of disconnect from society, which can feel impossible to fix.

Find Out Your Chronotype

Chronotype Spotter

It is relatively simple to know the best time for you to go to bed at night and get up in the morning. Use the Chronotype Spotter to help you identify your natural rhythm. Of course, the data you collect can only be reliable if you are not drinking coffee, caffeinated tea, or energy drinks. Start with one week and try to extend it to a longer period to get more accurate data. You can find this Chronotype Spotter with all the other worksheets in the printable workbook that is available for download at allonZcoaching.com/sleepitoff (use password SLEEP_IT_OFF).

Every day, for one or two weeks, record the time in the morning when you feel ready to tackle the most work or when you feel the most energized and motivated.

Because many of us are also wired for a midday nap, track the time of the day when you feel a dip in your energy level and a strong desire to take a nap around lunchtime – whether it is before or after lunch.

At the end of the day, write the time when you start feeling sleepy and wish you could go to bed for the night. Make sure it is not linked to your activity, though. For example, if every night at 6:30 pm you are on the bus and feel sleepy commuting after a long day of work, the bus might have something to do with your sleepiness. In this case, see what happens on days when you don't do this sleep-inducing activity. Write the time every single day for a couple of weeks and look at your chart to see whether there is a trend.

Tracking these three things for about two weeks gives you a better idea of what your ideal schedule is. I also suggest that you record your wake-up time and your bedtime. Doing so provides valuable information. For instance, you can find out how far away your bedtime is from the actual time when you start feeling tired at night. In the morning, you might notice that your energy peak is just minutes after you wake up in the morning and that actually, you lose this opportunity to take on important projects because you are having breakfast or are getting ready for the day.

In the example below, you can see that the subject goes to bed pretty late compared to when their body feels naturally tired. If they could advance their bedtime a bit, they would most likely benefit: they would sleep better and feel more refreshed in the morning.

Tracking how you sleep is a commitment, and for many people, not drinking caffeine for two weeks seems like an impossible challenge. If that's the case for you, start with a few days of tracking and see if you observe a pattern. It is essential to know that if you are struggling with sleep, caffeine intake is most likely making things worse. If you commit to improving your sleep, you might have to give it up, at least for a while. Also, keep in mind that if you are used to having caffeine every day, even just a bit, the first few days after you stop drinking it might not give you relevant tracking because you might often feel exhausted during the day and you might not experience any burst of energy for several days. If that is the case, allow for about a week before your body goes back to normal and you can record accurate information.

Chronotype Spotter

Example

TIME	Friday	Saturday	Sunday	...
Wake-up at...	6:15 am	8:30 am	8 am	
Alarm or Natural	Alarm	Natural	Natural	
Highest energy before noon at...	8:15 am	8:30 am	8 am	
Urge for nap at...	2:15 pm	none	2 pm	
Nap: YES or NO	No	No	No	
Natural desire to sleep after 6 pm	8:30 pm	9 pm	8:30 pm	
Actual Bedtime	10 pm	11:30 pm	10 pm	
Notes:	Felt rested in the morning	Bad dream + agitated (heavy meal?)	Took forever to fall sleep (cocktail & wine?)	

Chronotype Spotter

Download online

Track your sleep for at least one week while reporting below.

TIME	Friday	Saturday	Sunday	Monday	Tuesday	Wednesday	Thursday
Wake-up at...							
Alarm or Natural							
Highest energy before noon at...							
Urge for nap at...							
Nap: YES or NO							
Natural desire to sleep after 6 pm							
Actual Bedtime							
Notes:							

Staycation / Vacation Experiment

If tracking your sleep with the Chronotype Spotter doesn't seem appealing to you or if you feel like your daily routine makes it impossible, here is another option for you. Next time you are on vacation, quit coffee a week before and stay off it for the whole duration of your break. Follow your natural sleep cycle for as long as possible. That means going to bed as soon as you start feeling sleepy, and not setting the alarm for the next day. Try to wake up naturally for as long as you do the test, so that you follow your natural tendencies. Do that for the entire duration of the staycation or vacation.

This strategy can be challenging to apply. It is hard to follow our natural needs and go to bed as soon as we feel sleepy; we are not used to listening to our body this way. This test can give you a lot of knowledge about your natural sleep needs, even though it won't give you any information about a potential midday slow down. If you wish to pursue the vacation method, you can record the data in the Vacation Experiment worksheet.

Vacation Experiment
Example

	Friday	Saturday	Sunday	Monday	...
Natural Bedtime	9:15 pm	10:00 pm	10 pm	10 pm	
Natural Wake-up time	9:15 am	7:30 am	7 am	7 am	
Hours awake at night	1 hour	30 min	30 min	30 min	
Total hours slept	11 hours	9 hours	8.5 hours	8.5 hours	
Notes:	Was exhausted from trip	Slept well but tired after lunch	Good energy all day	Yoga and run felt good	

Vacation Experiment

Download online

Quit coffee and other caffeinated beverages a few days before your start tracking.
Stay off caffeine while filling out this log.

Follow your natural sleep cycle.

Go to bed as soon as you start feeling sleepy after 6 pm, and don't set an alarm for the next day.
Try to wake up naturally for as long as you do this experiment.

	Friday	Saturday	Sunday	Monday	Tuesday	Wednesday	Thursday
Natural Bedtime							
Natural Wake-up time							
Hours awake at night							
Total hours **slept**							
Notes:							

Morning/Evening Questionnaire (MEQ)

If you don't want to or don't feel that it is realistic for you to go through this testing phase to find out your chronotype, you can use the Morning/Evening Questionnaire developed by Horne and Östberg. It will help you find out whether you are an early bird or a night owl. A user-friendly version of that questionnaire has been created by the Australian Sleep Health Foundation. You can access it directly on their website.[8]

Ideally though, if you want to get in tune with your body and understand your sleep needs better, I recommend that you track your sleep and figure out your chronotype using the Chronotype Spotter or the Vacation Experiment worksheet first. Later on, you can fill out the questionnaire to compare the results. This is what I did, and the test results were spot on with my personal observations.

Assess Your Sleep Needs

After identifying when we need to sleep, we also need to find out how long we need to sleep. I recommend that you work on answering this question at the same time as filling out the Chronotype Spotter because, to get that information, you also need to be off daytime crutches such as coffee, energy drinks, caffeinated soda, or caffeinated tea.

With sleep, there is no one-size-fits-all, and some people need seven hours while others need nine hours. Some people need to sleep through the night, and others are wired to wake up once or twice, just like certain people are meant to take a nap while others don't. If you are not using crutches to stay alert – such as coffee or energy drinks – and feel healthy and rested every morning, chances are you are actually not sleep-deprived, even if you only sleep seven hours or if you sleep in two shifts each night.

Here are a few ways for you to find out how many hours of sleep you need each night.

During Your Vacation

When you are going through the Vacation Experiment, not only can you discover your chronotype, but you can also learn how many hours of sleep you need each night to feel fully rested since your goal is to wake up naturally every morning. This is valuable information to have if you want to work efficiently on improving your sleep. Of course, you might wake up naturally and still be exhausted in the morning. If that is your case, you will need to dig deeper. We will come back to this later.

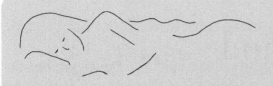

STORYTIME

Ryan knew how important good sleep is. He had been raised this way. He had always made sure he would get eight hours of sleep each night. But lately, he'd found it harder to sleep that long. At first, he found it difficult to sleep through the night and would always wake up before his alarm clock. But after a while, it also became hard for Ryan to fall asleep in the evening. He was so focused on getting his eight hours of snooze each night that it was creating a lot of stress for him. Soon, the fear of not sleeping enough started keeping him from sleeping.

Together, we decided to use one of Ryan's vacations as an opportunity to let go of the eight-hour obsession. He tracked his sleep to assess how many hours he actually needed to feel good. Interestingly, he found that 7 hours and 15 minutes were sufficient. Knowing that allowed him to lessen his fixation on the number eight, and after just a few weeks, it became clear that Ryan was getting enough sleep almost every single night now that he wasn't worrying so much about falling asleep. The stress was gone, and he felt refreshed and sharp again in the morning, ready for a long day of coding.

Tracking your sleep during a cherished and hard-earned vacation may not seem desirable to you because listening to your body's needs requires effort and discipline. Tackling the problem in a profound way can be life-changing, though, and is definitely worth it, I promise you!

Keep in mind that when you do the Vacation Experiment, you might not get very accurate results at first because you might have to catch up on some lost sleep. But once you are rested, you should be able to identify when you need to go to bed and when you need to wake up to feel your best.

Incremental Method

Many people don't get a vacation or might not have an entire week off at a time. Another way to identify how many hours of sleep you need is to go to bed 15 minutes earlier each night until you wake up naturally.

Let's imagine that right now you have to wake up at 6 am for work and usually fall asleep around 11 pm. Start going to bed earlier every night so you can fall asleep at 10:45 the first night, the following night at 10:30 pm, and so on until you end up falling asleep at a time that allows you to wake up at 6 am without an alarm.

Incremental Method

Download online

To define how long you need to sleep, you can either:

1/ Go to bed at a specified time and find out how late you need to sleep in the morning in order to wake up naturally and refreshed.

OR

2/ Decide on a specific wake-up time and find out when you need to go to bed at night in order to wake up naturally and refreshed at the pre-defined wake-up time.

	Bedtime	Natural Wake-up Time
Friday		
Saturday		
Sunday		
Monday		
Tuesday		
Wednesday		
Thursday		

This method has its pros and cons. It is convenient because you don't need a vacation to do the test. But the problem is if you are a night owl, you might not fall asleep early enough to ever wake up naturally, depending on your work or life schedule.

Some of us don't need to get up early and instead need to stay up late at night. Still, it is possible to do that same test. Just go to bed at your usual time and see when you wake up without an alarm.

If you decide to use the incremental method to define how many hours of sleep you need in order to wake up naturally and feel rested, you can use the Incremental Method worksheet shown on the next page. As with all the worksheets from this book, you can find it at allonZcoaching.com/sleepitoff. Use the password SLEEP_IT_OFF to download your workbook.

How to Accommodate Your Biological Patterns

It is not always realistic to live in harmony with our chronotype. Yet it is often possible to make some changes that can at least improve the situation. Even if you only add 15 minutes of good-quality sleep to your current nights, it could add up and make an enormous difference in the long term. If we put it in perspective, 15 minutes every night is almost two hours per week! It is over 90 hours of sleep each year, or about 11 extra nights.

Tired Too Early in the Evening

Some people – especially as they get older – need to go to bed so early that it might be difficult for them to meet their sleeping needs without feeling alienated. Going to bed at 7 pm can make you feel that you are missing out a lot. These people often go to bed later than their body would prefer. Still, since their body is also programmed to wake up super early in the morning, they cannot get their seven to nine hours of recommended sleep and soon end up sleep-deprived.

If this is you and it is hard for you to stay awake after 7 pm, it is crucial that you try to expose yourself to daylight in the later hours of the day as much as possible. This way, your body understands that it is not yet night time. Doing this routinely might help "recalibrate" your biological clock. You can, for instance, go for a brisk evening walk every single day while it is still bright outside, or plan an outdoor workout later in the day rather than early in the morning.

The idea here is to keep your body from wanting to sleep too early at night.

Once you go to bed, make sure your bedroom is dark, cool, and silent, so you won't be awakened too early in the morning by daylight, heat, or noise since it is already your natural tendency to wake up at the crack of dawn. Light is especially important in these cases: you want your body to think it is night time for as long as possible in the morning so that you get all the sleep you need.

Can't Wake Up in the Morning

For some people, especially teenagers, the biological clock is set up to get the body ready for sleep much later.[9] They can't fall asleep at night, and as a result, they wake up much later and struggle not to fall back asleep.

If you have teens at home, you are probably very familiar with this problem. This issue could be much smaller if they did not make the problem worse by exposing themselves to technology and screens later in the day. Parents of teens, why not have your adolescent read this chapter? I have three teens at home, and this is a recurring discussion we have.

If you tend to fall asleep late and be so exhausted in the morning that you want to sleep until noon, here are a few suggestions to keep you from aggravating the problem.

- No screen or technology after dinner, or at least for two or three hours before what feels like a reasonable bedtime for you;
- Keep all your devices off and out of your bedroom;
- Make sure your room is cool, dark, and quiet. Use blackout curtains, crack open the window if possible, use the appropriate bedding;
- Make sure nothing in your bedroom is screaming for you to be active. Keep your bedroom for sleeping only so you are not tempted to do things when you are trying to sleep;
- Take a stroll at night when it gets dark to help your body temperature go down and get your eyes and brain to register the decrease in daylight;
- Expose yourself to daylight as soon as possible when you get up every single morning, so your body and brain get the message that it is time to wake up and stay alert. During the wintertime, look into purchasing a light therapy lamp so you don't have to wait until the sun rises to be exposed to "sunlight."
- Be as physically active during the day as possible, especially in the morning and, if possible, outdoors, to help your system understand the different expectations you have for day and night.

If you look at this list, you probably notice that most of our teens are doing the opposite of what's recommended. Though teens have a shift in their biological clocks, the effects would be less of an issue if they did not engage in behavior that exacerbates the problem.[10]

Peer pressure and social media don't make it easy for them to turn off their phones and go to bed early. However, it is still worth educating them as much as possible on the topic.

What about the Elderly?

I have worked with many older people who thought they were sleep-deprived but, in fact, were not. How does this happen? It is commonly said that we need to sleep for eight hours every night. The people who wake up every night once or twice, or sleep only seven hours per night, start believing that there is something wrong with their sleep habits, even if they feel energized and well-rested throughout the day.

Though adults need less sleep than children and teens, research suggests that our sleeping needs remain pretty much the same through adulthood, no matter how old we are. And yet, older adults don't have the same sleeping pattern as younger adults, and they often complain about not sleeping well or enough, and waking up throughout the night or too early in the morning.

When it comes to sleep, several changes arise for seniors. After a certain age, hormone production goes down, which might lead to difficulties sleeping.[11] It does not mean that seniors need less sleep, but rather that they are not as well equipped to sleep anymore. It is a little like exercise. As we age, we don't need less exercise per se, but we have less strength and often less

DID YOU KNOW?

In a radio interview from January 2019 on France Inter, on the French national public radio, Dr. Patrick Lemoine, French psychiatrist and author, tells us about a study in which the sleep patterns of all members of a modern-day hunter-gatherer tribe in northern Tanzania were studied.[12] Older people were the ones who didn't sleep well during the night, compared to the rest of the tribe. Not only were they waking up very early, but their sleep was interrupted regularly. Lemoine suggests that this might be linked to the fact that while all the other members of the tribe had good reasons to sleep well (children need to grow, pregnant women need to provide for their babies, younger adults have to recharge to be alert while carrying out their daily activities for the tribe, etc.), the elderly didn't need as much energy and alertness during the day and thus could watch over the rest of the tribe at night. Hence, their poor sleep (France Inter 2019). This story was also mentioned in an article in *The Guardian*.[13]

energy to work out the way we did when we were 20. Talking about exercise, older adults are not usually as physically active during the day as their younger counterparts, which leads to more difficulty sleeping and sometimes also a lower need for recovery and rest.

Seniors also spend more time in the light stages of sleep rather than in the deep stages. As a result, they wake up more easily throughout the night. They don't sleep as deeply and might wake up feeling that they are not rested because they have spent too little time in the restorative stage of sleep and have been waking up regularly.

The overall health of older adults is also key. Seniors might have illnesses and take medications that interfere with sleep and sleep quality. Furthermore, as their muscle tone naturally decreases, their throat might become more easily obstructed, which might lead to disturbing snoring and sleep apnea.

It is essential to keep in mind that seniors often go to bed early compared to middle-aged adults, though. As a result, they wake up very early the next day and have the feeling that they don't sleep as long as they used to. In reality, many older people just start their night much earlier than before but still get the same amount of sleep.

HORMONES

If you are wondering why your sleep used to be a no-brainer and why things have changed, it might have to do with hormones, especially melatonin and cortisol. Our biological clock regulates our entire hormonal system.

Hormones act as chemical signals, and they trigger all kinds of effects on our body. Our hormonal system is complex, and for us to feel good, sleep well, and perform well intellectually, emotionally, and physically, we need our hormones to be in balance. It is important to understand that hormones are neither good nor bad. What is good is when they are present in the right amounts, and what is bad is when our hormones are out of balance.

Though our quality of sleep is impacted by our entire hormone system, there are four hormones that play a particularly significant role.

Melatonin

Without melatonin, we can't fall asleep or stay asleep. Production of melatonin – the hormone that tells our body when it is time to get ready for sleep – is linked to our biological clock. When our natural rhythm is not respected, not only do sleep issues arise, but we also struggle to wake up and stay alert during the day.

For our system to produce melatonin, our eyes need to detect a lack of light. In other words, we need to be in the dark. Melatonin production is also linked to lower body temperature.

Serotonin

Serotonin is the precursor to melatonin, and without it, we can't produce melatonin. Melatonin is directly proportional to serotonin, so the more serotonin we release during the day, the more melatonin we can produce at night. Although we are more used to associating endorphins with physical activities, we also release

DID YOU KNOW?
Some cells in our eyes are not used for vision at all. They are only used to regulate our sleep, informing our biological clock of the way it should adjust itself to the outside time and light. It is essential to know that artificial light does not seem to have the same effect on our body. According to a study by Ivy Cheung from the University of Illinois, natural light helps regulate our biological clock. In contrast, artificial light and lights from our screens seem to mess up our internal clock.[14] (Impact of Windows and Daylight Exposure on Overall Health and Sleep Quality of Office Workers: A Case-Control Pilot Study) This is why it is so important to spend as much time as possible outdoors or by the window if you have sleep issues, and even more so if you spend your day in an environment where light is artificial.

serotonin when we exercise, not just endorphins.[15] This is another reason why being physically active during the day is key to sleeping better. Besides, serotonin is more commonly known as the "happy chemical" because it largely contributes to happiness and well-being.[16] Serotonin regulates our mood. If we are serotonin-deficient, we often feel depressed, aggressive, and irritable, and we have trouble sleeping since we aren't able to produce the necessary amounts of melatonin. The resulting lack of sleep makes our moodiness and sadness worse, and from here, it becomes a vicious cycle. Serotonin is also recognized as the "self-esteem hormone."[17] We produce it when we feel appreciated and when our self-esteem is high, which makes it evident that when we have trouble sleeping, a holistic approach is necessary. We need to take into consideration our mental, emotional, social, and physical well-being, rather than focusing only on the mechanism of sleep. It is essential to concentrate on improving the quality of our days rather than being solely concerned with the time we spend in bed.

Cortisol

Cortisol is commonly known as the stress hormone and is produced when we are under stress, whether it is physical or emotional. For instance, if we work out intensely, our cortisol levels will go up. That is what we call physical stress. Emotional stress is triggered either by positive events, such as planning a wedding or a family vacation, or by negative thoughts such as those around a breakup, financial insecurity, or pressure at work. "People can experience tremendous stress in the workplace when they don't feel like they are part of the tribe. In today's world, our body is most likely to release cortisol in response to a threat to our ego, rather than a physical threat. This stress negatively affects cognitive ability, productivity, and importantly the ability to get a good night's sleep," says certified Executive and Performance Coach, Jill Avey.[18]

DID YOU KNOW?

We are not wired to sleep all night and be awake all day. We experience a dip in our cortisol and level of alertness around six hours after we wake up (often around lunchtime). If we are well-rested and have an active and enjoyable day, we might not even notice it. But if we are tired already, this dip in cortisol levels is very noticeable and might require a nap, even more so if what we are doing is not engaging. Who hasn't experienced the irresistible urge to close their eyes during a boring meeting? Often, we grab a sugary snack or an energy drink to combat this drowsiness.

If we work on lowering our stress, whether chronic or temporary, we can lower our cortisol level and, as a result, influence the quality of our sleep. Cortisol is released in different quantities, depending on whether our body decides that it is time to wake up (higher levels of cortisol) or go to sleep (lower levels of cortisol).

Cortisol usually has a terrible reputation because we often think of stress as being negative. It is important to remember that cortisol also gives us energy and makes us feel enthusiastic. Eagerness and excitement are also stress, but in a positive form. Cortisol, just like other hormones, is only bad if we have too much of it and too often. It is vital to have cortisol every day. For example, if we didn't have an increased release of cortisol in the morning, it would make it very hard for us to wake up and stay awake. If our levels of cortisol are too high at night, it also makes it very hard to relax and fall asleep.

Oxytocin

Oxytocin is another hormone that is directly involved in our sleep. Oxytocin is released when there is positive sensory stimulation: massage, a pleasant smell, sex, etc. Often referred to as the "love hormone" because its level goes up during an orgasm or while cuddling, oxytocin plays a vital role in our sleep. It acts as the counter hormone to cortisol by calming us down. It does this by not only lowering our blood pressure but also by bringing down our cortisol levels.[19] According to Carol Rinkleib Ellison, a clinical psychologist in Loomis, California, oxytocin "leaves you feeling tranquil and loving, and certainly that helps our path to sleep."[20]

Understanding the role of our hormonal system helps us realize that, to improve our sleep, it is critical to look at our quality of life. Do we have a life that promotes the secretion of these sleep-inducing hormones, or do we just go from one stressor to another? Oxytocin is crucial if we want to lower our cortisol. That is why things such as hugging, being with people we love, or getting a massage are all parts of a strategy to improve our sleep.

Most of the time, our sleep issues come from our activities during the day, so it is important to do things that help bring our body to where it should be when it is time to go to bed. Focusing on our nights is vital to begin this journey, but if we want to get results, we have to work on the quality of our days. Not only can it improve our sleep biologically, but it might also take our attention away from the problem itself and shift it toward a solution. Being hung up on our sleep issues can lead to chronic insomnia, but spending more energy on optimizing our days can help us avoid this problem.

Many people have trouble sleeping all year long, but when they are on vacation, they sleep "like babies." This is often because of a lack of stress the previous day, as well as a lack of stress while anticipating the next day. Taking our attention away from poor sleep and focusing on enjoying the day can help you improve your sleep. It is

 DID YOU KNOW?
Against all the odds, sex can be a marvelous way to sleep better. You might think that being aroused will keep you awake, but in fact, what happens hormonally while having sex is sleep-promoting, especially if you reach an orgasm. Having consensual and enjoyable sex helps boost the release of oxytocin and, as a result, helps your cortisol level. Orgasm also leads to the release of prolactin. This hormone makes your entire body and your mind feel relaxed and sleepy. How you reach your orgasm is entirely your choice, but keep in mind that when you feel jittery, and your mind is racing at night, having an orgasm might be way more efficient than reaching for a pill of melatonin.

a shift in mindset that we don't always think of, and that might not happen overnight, but it is important to work towards it as it is instrumental to our success.

Understanding the fundamentals of sleep is critical if you want to implement changes that have a genuine impact. Whether it is the need for brain waves to slow down, the strong link between the internal clock and sleep patterns, or the hormones involved in sleep, knowing how sleep works is the only way you can make changes that will matter and get results, whether you decide to fix your sleep on your own or with the guidance of a doctor, counselor, or coach.

Now that you understand the mechanics of sleep, let's dive a little deeper so you get a clear picture of the five key elements that are required for us to sleep well. Identifying these elements and knowing how they interact with each other will help you see why your sleep might be broken and how to fix it.

CHAPTER FOUR
Five Keys to Good Sleep

I have slept like a baby in the trunk of my SUV; I have had beautiful dreams on my daughter's bedroom floor; and when there was too much going on in the house, I have even slept like a log in the garage under the ping-pong table. I know what you think: no, I was not drunk! Sleeping on a pile of rock would most likely be no issue for me, as long as I could be confident that no one would bother me. But if someone so much as breathes or shifts next to me, I will wake up in a heartbeat and toss and turn the rest of the night. Am I a light sleeper? Yes, and no. Many people can't sleep if their room is not dark, but I can. Many people can't sleep if they are not in their bed, but I can. On the other hand, the faintest sound or smell will completely ruin my sleep. It doesn't mean that I need perfect silence to sleep. I have fallen asleep on the bleachers while attending a Deep Purple concert, and I can sleep through a Star Wars movie from beginning to end.

I have a weak spot when it comes to sleep, and you will soon understand which one it is when you read this chapter. There are five prerequisites that we need to fulfill if we want to fall asleep and sleep through the night. If one of these conditions is not met, we will struggle with sleep, no matter what we do. Some of us have no problem at all meeting the five requirements. Others struggle with a couple of them. And a rare few find it hard to meet any of them.

Understanding these key elements of sleep is critical to your being able to take action and improve your sleep. Let's review them now.

KEY #1: TIME FOR SLEEPING

One seemingly obvious but often overlooked requirement is to allocate seven to nine hours to sleep. If we don't set aside time to sleep, there is no way we can get the amount of rest we need. Sleep and recovery need to be near the top of our priority list. This is the number one mistake most people make, and this is the one I was consciously and proudly making for many years. Take a moment to ask yourself how often, in the past week, you felt tired and said to yourself, "I'll go to bed as soon as I am done with this." How often do you plan on going to bed but catch yourself doing some last-minute chores, checking social media one last time, or prepping some quick snacks for the next day? How much time goes by between the moment you decide to go to bed and the moment you find yourself actually in bed and falling asleep? Which tasks, chores, or habits systematically take priority over going to sleep? It seems to me that crumbs on the countertop are more important to us than sleep; Facebook likes are more important to us than sleep; folded underwear is more important to us than sleep, and the list goes on.

KEY #2: ACCUMULATION OF TIREDNESS

During our waking hours, our body accumulates sleep-promoting molecules called hypnogenic molecules. These sleep-promoting molecules are released all day long while we are awake, and the amount released depends on how active our brain is. Once enough of these hypnogenic molecules have built up in our body, we get sleepy. During the night, our brain activity decreases, and so does the production of hypnogenic molecules. Our stores eventually deplete as the night progresses, and we wake up once none are left.[1]

Exercise Can Help!

High levels of physical activity can help us fall asleep at night because exercise increases the production of a hypnogenic molecules in our body.[2] For instance, adenosine is a sleep-promoting molecule that is produced when we exercise.[3]

The necessity to build up adenosine and other hypnogenic molecules during the day is an important fact to take into consideration when you try to get more sleep. You need to be tired enough to fall asleep. If you don't feel tired but still go to bed earlier to sleep longer, you also need to add extra physical activity into your day. Otherwise, you don't give your body a chance to accumulate enough hypnogenic hormones during the shorter day, and it is very hard for you to fall asleep.

If the life we live during the day doesn't allow us to accumulate enough adenosine, it will affect our sleep negatively. This is why many people who have trouble falling asleep at night might see their problems worsen when they get an opportunity to sleep in later in the morning.

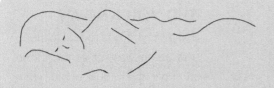

STORYTIME

When Michael started working with me, he had been struggling with sleep for years. He would quickly fall asleep on his couch every night watching sports on TV, but once he made it to bed, he would toss and turn for hours, eyes wide open. TV helped him forget all about work and his bad-tempered manager. Unfortunately, falling asleep in front of the TV would halt the production of hypnogenic molecules and deplete his stores. Once Michael made it to his bed, he didn't have enough to fall asleep again. He was not only tired; his blood sugar levels were creeping up, as was his blood pressure. At 62, he knew he was at risk for type 2 diabetes and cardiovascular disease.

Together, we thought outside the box and figured out other ways to unwind at night that would allow him to fall asleep in bed. He ended up alternating audiobooks and relaxing podcasts that he could listen to in bed. He would fall asleep just the same, but this time in his bed. He also programmed white noise so that the sudden silence would not wake him up once his "show" was over. Improving his sleep made him realize that he had the power to improve his health. He decided to work on his eating habits too and greatly improved his general health.

Even if you don't struggle with sleep regularly, this tip can still be useful. I have worked with many clients who slept well all week but could not fall asleep on Sunday nights. They were convinced it was the stress of going back to work the next morning that kept them from relaxing. For a few of them, that was true. But for many, the actual culprit was sleeping in on Sunday morning, which gave them less time to accumulate hypnogenic molecules and kept them from being tired enough to fall asleep come nighttime.

Keeping the length of our days regular is very important to accumulate enough sleep-inducing molecules to fall asleep. Therefore, I recommend that people establish a consistent bedtime schedule and stick to it as much as possible, including on the weekend.

KEY #3: HARMONY WITH BIOLOGICAL CLOCK

Our biological clock is a major player when it comes to regulating our sleep. If we don't align our sleep schedule with our internal clock and our circadian rhythm, things usually don't go well. Again, some of us are more flexible than others. Still, if sleep is an issue for you, it might be impossible to improve your sleep if you keep trying to force your body to go against your internal clock.

An excellent way to see the importance of our biological clock is to consider something like jet lag or daylight saving. It can be tough to fall asleep when we travel through different time zones or when we have to go to bed an hour earlier because of daylight saving. Even a one-hour time change can make a tremendous difference in the way we fall asleep and in the way we feel during the day. So, if every night, you go to bed a couple of hours earlier or later than what your biological clock tells you, imagine the effects that it might have on your body, even though you have gotten used to it and have settled for it! Of course, we have constraints, and we don't always have a say when it comes to our bedtime. But

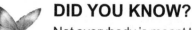

DID YOU KNOW?
Not everybody is meant to sleep the same way, or at the same time. Waking up in the middle of the night, for example, might not be an issue for some people. According to Roger Ekirch, History Professor at Virginia Tech, Europeans in pre-industrial times used to stay awake for extended periods in the middle of the night rather than sleep through the night. This is what he calls "segmented sleep" and is equivalent to sleeping our nights in two shifts rather than one.[4]

being aware of the problem and knowing what our body needs can help us take steps in the right direction.

Even though our biological clock is part of our genetic makeup, we have some influence on it. Our body is sensitive to external factors that help our biological clock adjust to the actual time on our watch. There are two key factors involved in the setting of our biological clock. The first one is the alternation between daylight and darkness. Indeed, our body is wired to be active during the day and asleep during the night. The second key factor is our core body temperature. When our core temperature goes up, our metabolism increases so that we are wide awake and able to perform. When our body temperature goes down, our metabolism slows down, which allows us to fall asleep. [5, 6] It is like a mini hibernation. We will elaborate later on those two factors and how we can use them to improve our sleep.

Adjusting our internal clock to accommodate our schedule is not the easiest task. To some extent, we do it when we travel and change time zones. Think of it as if every single cell in our body has its own biological clock. This is one reason why when we are jet-lagged, we don't just feel sleepy at the wrong time. Many of us also feel hungry at the wrong time.

KEY #4: MELATONIN RELEASE

As mentioned before, light and body temperature are both involved in our sleep process,[7] and a combination of darkness and the right core body temperature helps our body and mind to relax, get ready for sleep, and produce melatonin, also called the "sleep hormone."[8]

One thing that prevents melatonin production is keeping our body temperature too high near the end of the day. This can happen when we work out right before bedtime, or if our extremities are cold in the evening and our body raises its core temperature to compensate. Sleeping with socks might not sound appealing, but it can help increase your production of melatonin. This is also why most people find it easier to fall asleep in a cool room.

Another factor affecting our production of melatonin is light, especially blue light, which comes from the sun but also from televisions and the screens of computers, tablets, and phones. When we expose ourselves to blue light, we produce less melatonin. So, if you are getting your phone out as soon as you wake up in the morning, that isn't an issue at all. Indeed, checking your phone right when you get up in the morning might help your body wake up. Unfortunately, it can have the same effect at night. If you bring your technology into your room and check your emails or social media right before bed (or when you wake up during the night), the blue light might slow your melatonin production and you could have trouble falling (back) to sleep. No judgment, no blaming, and 100% understanding, believe me! Though it may be very tempting or sometimes necessary to expose ourselves to blue light before bed, we must remind ourselves that these habits have a substantial impact on the quality of our sleep.

When blue light from the sun diminishes, melatonin production rises, leading to the onset of sleep. But if we replace blue light from the sun with blue light from electronic devices, we are disrupting the process that would otherwise allow us to fall asleep. Not all electronic devices are made equal, though. E-readers, such as the original Kindle, don't represent as big a problem as backlit tablets or smart phones, since they do not shine light directly into the eyes of the reader. By the same token, using a night lamp with a dim warm light to read a paper book or a magazine won't be as disruptive as using a tablet, especially if you use a red bulb.

At the same time as daylight fades, our core body temperature starts dropping during the evening, and it will stay low for the rest of the night before slowly rising in the morning.

It is essential to sleep in a dark, cool room so that melatonin production can peak around 3 or 4 am when both light and temperature are at their minimum. Our bedding also needs to be comfortable and not cause our body to overheat.

Here are a few elementary steps you can take right away to increase your melatonin production:

- No screens after dinner (or at least for one to two hours before bedtime) and no screen in your bedroom
- Dim lighting in the house for at least two hours before bedtime
- A calming and refreshing stroll in the dark or around sunset to show your body that it is dark outside and also to cool down a bit (no speed walking!)
- Allowing your body's core temperature to go down naturally. Don't dress too warmly for the night, but make sure your extremities (head, hands, and feet) are not cold.

Many of us use our phones as an alarm, or sometimes to record our sleep, which means that we keep our phones under our pillows or on the nightstand. This will have many adverse effects on our sleep. Not only does it keep us from disconnecting from work and other daily activities, and inhibit our ability to relax and fall asleep, but it can also hinder melatonin release.

We might think, "Well, my phone is sitting next to my bed, but I am not using it." But let's be honest with ourselves for a moment and think about our nightly routine. I check my emails one last time before turning the lights off, don't you? I jump and answer a message whenever my phone vibrates before I've fallen asleep. I might have all the best intentions in the world, but there are nights when I forget to put my phone on airplane or do-not-disturb mode, and it pings, and I check it. Not to mention in the middle of the night, when I wake up and check the time. Sometimes I can't help but check my social media feed, really quick, while I am at it.

KEY #5: SLOW BRAIN WAVES

Screens, emails, and social media can be real disturbances in the sense that they keep us in a state of alertness that makes it impossible for our brains to slow down and fall asleep. Technology is not the only thing that can keep your brain waves from slowing down. Worries, anxiety, fear, heated discussions, excitement, anticipation, sexual arousal, noise, pain, poor digestion, etc. can be just as detrimental. Anything that requires attention can keep us awake.

Calm Down Sympathetic Nervous System

Our sympathetic nervous system is the nervous system that keeps us alert, whether for positive or negative reasons. It is also known as the "fight-or-flight" system. It maintains our brain activity and is linked to high levels of adrenaline, noradrenaline, glutamate, acetylcholine, cortisol, etc. To fall asleep, we need our brain waves to slow down, which means that we cannot be in a state of high alertness.

One factor that affects our sympathetic system is whether or not we feel safe. We might not feel safe from external physical attacks, or we might be feeling insecure because of our financial situation, our work, our relationships, our immigration status, etc. Therefore, we must assess our quality of life on a deep level if we want to sleep better. We must honestly address everything that goes on during the time we are awake – stress, eating habits, physical activity, happiness – rather than during the time we spend in bed.

Activate Parasympathetic Nervous System

Finding ourselves in a calmer state doesn't just mean that we have turned down our sympathetic system. It goes further than this, as we need our parasympathetic nervous system to have taken over and started releasing substances such as serotonin, melatonin, and gamma-aminobutyric acid (GABA) to slow down our brain waves.

GABA is not a hormone, like serotonin or melatonin. It is an amino acid we can find in fermented foods, such as yogurt, kefir, or tempeh, and in certain varieties of tea.[9] GABA is not an essential amino acid, though. This means that we also produce it naturally, without having to get it from our food. GABA is well-known as the main inhibitory neurotransmitter of the central nervous system. It reduces communication between the cells in our brain and nervous system. As a result, it has a tremendous impact on our ability to slow down mental activity and relax for the night.[10]

Night exposure to light in general, and blue light in particular, impacts your sleep negatively. Even if your device is set to "night light" (the setting that screens blue light out and only lets red light through), checking your phone activates the parts of your brain that should be sleeping. It activates your sympathetic system and keeps you from sleeping well because it raises your stress level, even if you don't feel stressed.

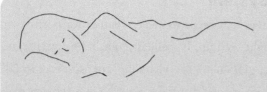

STORYTIME

When Janet came to me, she was suffering from onset insomnia. It was hard for her to fall asleep at night. Since she had to wake up early for work every morning, she was becoming exhausted, finding it harder and harder to stick to her workout schedule, and had started to pile on extra pounds. She assumed that the problem was stress and that her new position was the culprit, even though she really liked her company and enjoyed her colleagues very much. She considered changing jobs but felt very torn because she enjoyed it and loved the benefits.

After doing a bit of digging, we realized that her sleep issues had all started after she'd been transferred to a new division within her company. She had been sleeping fine at the time, and only Sunday nights were problematic. She could never fall asleep and ended up exhausted on Monday mornings. She didn't worry about it until it became more frequent. What had started as a Sunday night issue was now her new normal.

We worked together on implementing some healthy eating habits, but it soon became clear that food changes were not what she needed to sleep well. Rituals didn't do much, either, until we had a breakthrough. We realized that since her transfer at work, she had started hanging out with her new colleagues regularly on Saturday nights. As a result, she slept in on Sundays, which was something new to her. On Sunday night, she had not accumulated enough tiredness to fall asleep (key #2). The frustration would build up, and she would worry about not performing well the next day. She would find it impossible to relax (key #5). Little by little, the fear of not falling asleep on other days of the week grew, and she started having issues falling asleep every single night.

Once we'd identified the mechanism that had broken her sleep, she knew that she could fix the original problem by waking up earlier on Sunday mornings and adding a long hike or a tennis game to her Sunday. That would not fix the problem right away, but knowing that she had a solution gave her the peace of mind she needed to relax other nights of the week. She made a few other minor adjustments to her routine, and within three months, she was able to sleep well again. If she had not identified that she was not accumulating enough tiredness on Sundays, she might never have fixed the problem. Improving her situation required patience and a few months of effort, but it was nothing compared to quitting a job and a team that she truly enjoyed.

So, even if you don't like the idea, one of the first steps you can take if you are having trouble sleeping is to not allow electronics in your bedroom. Which is more important to you: tracking your sleep with an app on your phone or sleeping? Being connected to your network 24/7 or resting and regenerating your body and mind while you sleep so you can have more meaningful connections during the day? And if you think you need your phone as an alarm, remember that not so long ago, we did not have smartphones and yet we all showed up at work on time every morning. You might be tired of my repeating that screens are sleep-killers. I have to, though, because this is something we don't want to acknowledge, and even if we hear it and read it everywhere, it doesn't seem to sink in. I plead guilty, too. Sometimes, I catch myself checking emails just before turning off the lights…

An excellent way to help activate your parasympathetic system is to establish nighttime rituals. Rituals are more intentional than a routine, and we put sense into our rituals. They have a purpose; they are not as mindless as habits can be. We often use rituals with babies such as a warm bath after dinner, a lullaby, a soft light once they lie down. When they get older, we still tuck them in, read them a story, review the good things that happened in their day, kiss them good night… We do this because we know how reassuring it is for them to know what's coming, to prepare, to ease into the "scary night" with a protocol that they know well and makes them feel secure. So why don't we use rituals for ourselves? We also need reassurance and a feeling of security. Bedtime rituals can help tremendously with that. Taking a stroll after dinner, keeping a journal, soaking in a warm bath – enriched or not with Epsom salts and essential oils – slipping into your favorite sweater, drinking a cup of milk, meditating. There is no right or wrong as long as the rituals you go for make sense to you and make you feel good while not interfering with good sleep. Eating a donut before bedtime or watching the news are probably not the best rituals to help you sleep!

To improve our sleep, we cannot just direct our attention on one of these requirements. Sleep won't happen unless all the requirements are met, and this is why a holistic approach is necessary. Sleep is a multifaceted phenomenon. If you do everything to be in agreement with your internal clock but are super stressed when you go to bed, sleep won't happen because your brain won't be able to slow down. If you are able to relax but are trying to sleep in a bright room just after reading a book on your back-lit tablet, chances are it won't work either because you won't release melatonin.

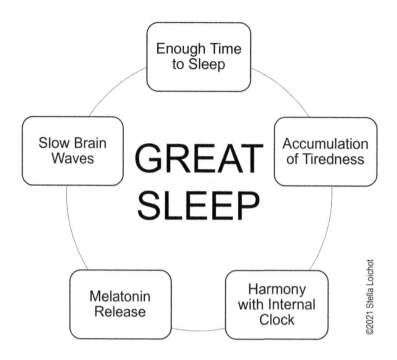

©2021 Stella Loichot

Some people are natural sleepers, which means that even if they have a very unhealthy lifestyle, they can still sleep perfectly fine because the five requirements are met no matter what. At the other extreme, some people need to pay very close attention to the five key principles described in this chapter because their body won't naturally do the work for them. It is very similar to the fact that some people can stay trim on a fried-chicken-with-mayo diet, while others seem to gain weight just by looking at a piece of chocolate cake. Life is not fair; we know it. Fortunately, when it comes to sleep, most of us don't struggle with all five prerequisites. If we are well informed and if we concentrate our efforts on what truly matters and on the conditions that are not met naturally by our body, we will experience the best results.

When I look back at the sleeping habits that lead to my collapse, it is evident that I was not allocating enough time for sleep (requirement one was not met). It was not an easy fix, but it was straightforward, and I tackled it right away. Now, there is another requirement that my body has trouble meeting. As explained before, I could sleep on a concrete floor but can't stand the flutter of a butterfly. What I struggle with the most is slowing down the activity in my mind. I am always on high alert. Not necessarily thinking or worrying but just on the lookout and vigilant (requirement five is not easily met). As a result, anything that my brain perceives as the slightest threat will wake me up. These "threats" can be as insignificant as a gentle click or a blinking light. It wouldn't be an issue if I could go back to sleep right away, but that rarely happens. Not only is it very hard for me to calm down again, but on top of it, once I have slept for a few minutes, I am not tired enough to fall back to sleep (requirement two is not met). It took me years to understand how I was wired and why it made my sleep so uneven. Now that I know the five essentials to good sleep and how they apply to my own needs, I have figured out many ways to protect my sleep. For instance, it is best for me to go to bed slightly later than usual if I know that I will be awakened within a couple of hours. When my teens go out, I will lose less sleep by waiting until they come home safely rather than falling asleep for a bit and waking up when I hear them come home. If I wake up, it ruins the night for me. It often happened before I took a more systematic approach to my sleep. It is also best for me to find a quiet place, no matter how uncomfortable or inconvenient it might seem, rather than try to sleep in a bed where I can expect some kind of disruption, whether it is the cat coming in, a spouse moving around, or the sound of the fridge in the kitchen.

When one or more of the five essentials is not met, whatever other efforts we make cannot pay off. This is why, to work efficiently on improving your sleep, you need first to identify which might be the requirement (or requirements) that you are not meeting regularly. All the strategies and tools presented in this book have the aim of helping you fulfill all five of the criteria for sleep. But if you want to see results without running out of juice, you first need to identify why your own sleep is broken.

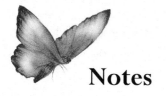

Notes

CHAPTER FIVE
Why Is Your Sleep Broken?

Just as there are five key factors involved in a sound sleep, there can be many reasons why someone is struggling with their sleep. More often than not, it is a combination of several elements. Besides the obvious ones, such as getting married or working night shifts, here is a list of common reasons for sleep deprivation:

- Depression or anxiety
- Psychological trauma (linked, for instance, to domestic or sexual abuse)
- Over-thinking and tending to keep emotions bottled up
- Perfectionism or an irrepressible need for total control
- Stress, whether it is positive (such as anticipation of a trip) or negative (financial distress, for instance)
- Physical issues such as chronic pain, gastric reflux, trouble breathing, illnesses
- Medication
- Specific sleeping disorders such as restless legs syndrome or sleep apnea
- Unhealthy lifestyle (poor eating habits, smoking, alcohol consumption)
- Unsuitable environment (too loud, too bright, too hot)

Sleep troubles fall into two categories: insomnia and parasomnia. Parasomnia is something undesirable that happens during our sleep, while insomnia is an inability to sleep in the first place and maintain sleep throughout the night.

INSOMNIA

Insomnia is defined by the Mayo Clinic as "a common sleep disorder that can make it hard to fall asleep, hard to stay asleep, or cause you to wake up too early and not be able to get back to sleep." Insomnia can be detrimental not only to your energy level and mood but also to your health, your level of performance at work, and, more generally, to the quality of your life.[1]

There are two types of insomnia: acute insomnia, which lasts only a few days or weeks, and chronic insomnia, which lasts for at least a month. Initially, the word insomnia meant "chronic inability to sleep."

About 30% of adults around the world have insomnia.[2] Women are more affected than men.[3]

We can compare insomnia to allergies, in the sense that, over time, smaller and smaller disturbances are needed to trigger an insomniac episode. What that means is that the first episode of insomnia might be caused by quite a stressful or traumatizing event – such as a divorce or money problems. But as people deal more often with insomnia, an argument or just the fear of not sleeping becomes enough to trigger a new episode. This phenomenon is one reason why working on improving our sleep is not a quick and easy process. Though it takes time, patience, and dedication, solving our sleep problems is within reach.

Common Causes for Insomnia

There are many reasons why people struggle with insomnia. Some of those reasons might seem easy to fix, while others are hard to spot.

For this book, I have decided to focus on the most common issues that adults deal with. Still, all the tools shared here can be applied to all kinds of situations. They can help you discover what your own issues are so that you can mitigate their effect on your quality of life.

Stress and Cortisol

Whether it is negative or positive, stress keeps us awake because it prevents our brain from slowing down. We often think of stress as something negative and unpleasant. Though being overworked, fighting with a partner, or worrying about climate change creates unpleasant stress, anticipation for things like weddings or vacations can be very pleasant. These events, even if they create stress that we enjoy, can still interfere with good sleep.

The fact that stress makes it difficult for us to fall asleep properly or to sleep well through the night is a genuine problem, not only because our lives are becoming more and more stressful but also because if we stress about our sleep, it can sometimes perpetuate insomnia.

It is common to go through a particularly stressful period of our life and thus develop insomnia. If we don't get too hung up on it, the problem often disappears after a few days or weeks, once the stressor itself has gone. But if we worry about the fact that we won't be able to perform well the next day, or that our health will suffer if we don't sleep enough, we might obsess and stress about our quality of sleep, and this can be enough to perpetuate our insomnia for months or years. That's how, often, an otherwise temporary insomnia episode turns into chronic insomnia, long after the initial reason for insomnia has disappeared. We end up not even remembering that there was a trigger in the first place. We think it has always been this way.

The fear of being sleep-deprived and not performing well the next day is common. If you suspect that it might be the problem, ask yourself the following questions:

- Do I sleep better when I am on vacation?
- Do I sleep better on the weekend?

If you answer yes to one or both questions, your insomnia could come from the pressure to perform well the next day. When you are on vacation, you might be reassured by the fact that you can take naps during the day to catch up on sleep if needed, or you simply won't feel the pressure to be well-rested the next day. This reassurance is sometimes enough to let you calm down and sleep.

Because of this, it is crucial not to worry about a few awful nights. It is also essential to have a plan to take care of the problem and feel confident that you can find a solution. When you want to improve your sleep, the first step is to work on everything else but your sleep: your food, your physical activity, your relationships, your work, etc. Once you make improvements in those areas of your life, sleep often improves. If we focus too much on the sleep we are not getting, we are usually contributing to a vicious cycle.

If you are not sleeping well, your first step is to identify which of the five requirements for sleep are not being met. The second step is to relax and start small by making your days healthier so that little by little, your nights also become healthier.

The idea here is that once you know how important sleep is, and you also know that you can sleep better, if you take your time, you can eventually fix your sleep. I have seen it happen many times! All along the process, though, it is important to keep in mind that, even though sleep should be a priority, having a terrible night or a few poor nights is usually not a big deal. It is the chronic aspect of poor sleep that is damaging to our body and to our health in the long run. Partying, being too stressed out, being too excited to fall asleep for a while, being sleep-deprived because we just gave birth to twins, etc. – that is not a problem. It might be tough, but it will not ruin your health as long as things stay temporary. Just like eating a decadent piece of cake won't jeopardize your waistline. Even binge eating for a week while you are on vacation shouldn't kill you, whereas overeating for a year without realizing it might put you at risk.

The first thing to do if you are having issues with sleep and sleep deprivation – after you have decided to take care of the problem and read this book – is to accept the fact that you are not sleeping well and go from there. There is a problem, that's how it is, and you can take care of it. There is no point in beating yourself up over it. Be very methodical and don't rush through the process of recovery. You can get results if you take your time and proceed step by step, using the ready-to-print workbook that is available for download at allonZcoaching.com/sleepitoff. Awareness and acceptance are an enormous part of the solution. Falling asleep and sleeping well require that we acknowledge the issue, accept the fact that we have the power to deal with it (no, we can't play the victim anymore), and then let go and relax, trusting that we have the skills to work through this, if we only take our time.

Depression and Anxiety

Mental health problems such as depression and anxiety are directly linked to insomnia. According to the National Sleep Foundation, people suffering from insomnia are 10 times more likely to have clinical depression and 17 times more likely to have anxiety.[4] When we are exhausted, our emotions are much harder to manage, but we also look at life differently and can't handle obstacles in the same way. If you feel sad on a regular basis and can't seem to be motivated enough to go through life the way you would like to, the quality of your sleep might be one reason.

Unfortunately, it also works the other way around. People who suffer from depression or anxiety are also much more likely to suffer from insomnia. Harvard Medical School explains in an article updated in 2019 that, although chronic sleep problems affect "only" 10 to 18% of the U.S. adult population, they affect 50 to 80% of patients in a typical psychiatric practice, especially those who suffer from depression or anxiety.[5]

If you tend to wake up very early in the morning and not be able to go back to sleep, depression might be the culprit.[6] Depression can be directly linked to what experts call sleep maintenance insomnia, which differs from sleep-onset insomnia. Sleep-onset insomnia is when you find it hard to fall asleep at night. Sleep maintenance insomnia translates into difficulty in staying asleep through the night or the inability to sleep long enough in the morning. As a general rule of thumb, younger people are often more affected by sleep-onset insomnia. In contrast, middle-aged and older adults often have to battle against sleep maintenance insomnia. In addition, certain antidepressant medications can interfere with sleep patterns and can make sleeping difficult.[7] It is critical that you talk to your health care provider about these issues and explore potential solutions and alternatives with them.

Pain

It is no secret that physical pain keeps us from sleeping well. We can't find a comfortable position to lie in, or we wake up often during the night, having to shift positions. It has been estimated that up to 60% of people suffering from chronic pain also have insomnia.[8]

The problem is that sleep deprivation makes it harder for us to manage pain, and it decreases our ability to recover from injuries that cause pain. Furthermore, when using opioid medication (painkillers) to reduce pain, it is essential to know that those medications might interfere with the quality of our sleep and lead to sleep deprivation and even more pain. Not only do opiates cause disturbances such as snoring and sleep apnea because they are respiratory depressants, but they also block access to deep sleep and REM sleep, which are the most restorative stages of sleep.[9]

This vicious cycle can make it hard to improve sleep quality and increase sleep duration. But not only does it make sleep even more valuable (and worth our time); we also see immediate improvements after making small changes, which usually turn the cycle into something positive.

Medication

We will address sleeping pills in the last chapter of the book, but it is important to know that when you take non-sleep medication, insomnia, sleep disorders, or just poor-quality sleep may all be side effects. Make sure you are talking about sleep with your health care provider and your pharmacist and that you are reading the information that comes with your meds.

Opioid pain medication can lead to disrupted sleep, but so can certain antidepressants.[10]

Any medication that contains caffeine will most likely harm your sleep. We often use these against headaches or migraines. Medications containing alcohol, such as cold, flu, and cough medicine, can also interfere with a good night's sleep. Medicines for high blood pressure might also keep you up at night, as well as drugs to boost a sluggish thyroid and those containing cortisone. They are often used in relation to arthritis, skin conditions, allergic reactions, and even certain cancers.

Nutrient Deficiencies

A deficiency of Vitamin D or magnesium might be one reason you have trouble sleeping. So, if sleep has been an issue for you, it is important to talk to your health care provider and run some blood work to make sure you don't have a nutrient deficiency.

For many of us, eating a healthy diet with a great variety of mostly plant-based foods is enough to provide us with all the required nutrients. Some people, however, need a supplement under the supervision of a doctor.

Eating Habits

Eating a healthy diet is far from easy for some of us. If this is the case for you, it is worth looking into getting help from a professional to improve your eating habits, which can vastly improve your sleep.

Digestion requires substantial effort from your body and produces a lot of energy and heat. We call this the thermogenic effect of food. If we eat a hard-to-digest meal, for instance with red meat, fried food, cheese, dessert, etc., chances are that we will wake up around 3 or 4 am, sweaty, hot, and most likely agitated and uncomfortable. Have you ever found yourself throwing off the covers after you have had a copious dinner? The thing is, we are aware of the effects that an extreme meal can have, so if we eat a double cheeseburger, followed by a large piece of cheesecake (I have done it many times!), we shouldn't be surprised to wake up in the middle of the night. Digestion can keep us from sleeping even if we don't have such an obviously heavy meal. Depending on our age, our metabolism, and many other factors, a small piece of chicken or apple pie might be all that's needed for us to stay awake.

Because my brain is so easily awakened by internal and external factors, I have to eliminate all potential disruptions if I want to get a good night's sleep. One thing I had to accept, to improve my sleep and piece myself back together, was that with age, some foods and beverages, that had no effect on my sleep before, have become my worst enemies. In my 20s, diet did not affect my sleep at all. Then, in my 30s, I could not eat lamb or beef for dinner or have several alcoholic beverages in the evening without risking a disrupted night. When I reached my early 40s, even chicken or a glass of wine became an issue. Now, I notice not only the effect of my dinner on the quality of my nights but also the effect of the food I eat during the day. I can only sleep well if I make sure that all day long, I am not exceeding the caloric needs of my body. Too much food compared to my physical activity, and I can bet on a short night's sleep. It doesn't mean that I am always controlling everything I eat or drink to sleep like a log. Sometimes I choose to indulge, even if I know that my rest will suffer. But I do so knowingly and can plan for the consequences. Life is about compromising and finding a satisfying balance. What's the point of sleeping well if our life is otherwise miserable?

It is essential to always keep an open mind as to what the reason for poor sleep could be and accept the fact that, with age, things rarely become easier and you must be very attuned to your body's needs. I have worked with many women whose sleep and hot flashes improved once they started establishing healthier eating behaviors, not just at night but all day long. We will talk about hot flashes and menopause in more detail in chapter eight. Many of my clients, no matter what gender they are, have seen their snoring diminish and their disruptive dreams vanish once they improved their eating habits.

Caffeine

Caffeine is not present only in coffee. There is caffeine in tea (but not in herbal tea), in soda, in energy drinks, and also in guarana. Guarana is a substance that is often added to energy drinks, and it contains four times the amount of caffeine that coffee has. Take a second look at the list of ingredients on your energy drinks because this chemical could make the difference between a good and a bad night.[11]

Caffeine is most effective within four to six hours of consumption, but it takes much longer for it to be completely cleared out of our system.[12] Caffeine can remain in your body for more than 12 hours, and it can affect your sleep for even longer. Research mentioned in the National Institutes of Health states that "ingestion of caffeine at a dose of 150 mg enhances cognitive performance for at least 10 hours."[13] One cup of brewed coffee contains about 100 mg of caffeine. One espresso has about 65 mg. An average cup of black tea contains about 50 mg of caffeine, while green tea has about 30 mg. The longer you let your tea steep, the more potent it will become.[14] Keep this in mind next time you have coffee with lunch or drink tea throughout the day and expect to be in bed by 9 pm. Indeed, another study revealed that consumption of caffeine within six hours of bedtime could reduce the total duration of sleep by up to one hour.[15]

Many of us are unconsciously addicted to caffeine, but we do not know how it works in our body.

About 80% of my clients have been drinking coffee every single day for many years, yet only 16% consider themselves addicted to caffeine. Most of them have never tried to quit coffee intentionally, but when, at some point in their life, coffee has not been available to them, they've had a glimpse of how hard life is without it.

Four times a year, I coach at a corporate wellness screening event, where I coach about 100 people as they get screened for various conditions. Guidelines for the screening are straight forward. To get their cholesterol level and blood sugar checked, people need to have fasted for at least nine hours. No food, no coffee, just water since the night before. Otherwise, they can't get the blood work done. These screening events usually run until noon, and though participants get hungry in the late morning, they rarely complain much because skipping breakfast is not an issue for them.

On the other hand, almost all of them struggle because of the lack of caffeine. For the majority, coffee is the very first thing they reach for after the screening is over. Until then, they can't think straight, they have no energy, and they get headaches. It is eye-opening to see so many people distressed by the lack of coffee while knowing that they don't acknowledge their addiction. Now, ask yourself: How do you feel about quitting coffee, tea, or caffeinated soda for one or two weeks?

I go without coffee for about 10 days two or three times per year. Sometimes, it is very easy. I sleep a little more, maybe have to take a few power-naps around lunchtime, but nothing dramatic. Other times – it has happened twice over the past five years – it is a horrible withdrawal experience. My entire body aches and all my muscles are sore; I have migraines for several days, I am exhausted, and I feel as though I could sleep 14 hours per day. When that happens, I know that I was long due for a break from caffeine. I don't drink colossal amounts of it anymore, but I drink it every day, and that's enough for me to become addicted. Since I don't like this feeling of dependence, taking breaks from caffeine gives me a sense of control, and it is like going through a detox. I feel clean and energized once the first few days of deprivation are over.

Do you know how caffeine really works?

As we use energy throughout the day, we consume ATP (adenosine triphosphate), and the by-product of this consumption is ADP (adenosine diphosphate). ADP is what tells our body that we are tired. We have receptors for ADP in our brain, and as ADP comes and attaches itself to those receptors, our brain gets the message "I am sleepy, I am tired, I need to rest." This is where caffeine comes into the picture. Caffeine will take the place of ADP on the ADP receptors and make those receptors unavailable. Caffeine will keep these receptors busy for hours but won't activate them and allow them to communicate the message to our brain that we are sleepy the way ADP would.

Caffeine doesn't give you a boost of energy. It doesn't remove fatigue. Caffeine simply keeps your brain from being informed that you are tired and sleep-deprived. As a result, you feel alert and energized. The effects of caffeine start between a few minutes to a couple of hours after you consume it and can last for many hours, depending on the person.

When someone drinks large quantities of coffee, it becomes a more severe problem. All the ADP receptors are occupied by caffeine molecules, and ADP has nowhere to go. As a result, once the effects of caffeine wear off and the caffeine has been processed, the ADP receptors are flooded by the ADP that has been waiting around, and the feeling of tiredness that results is irresistible. If that happens when you're in bed, it might not be such a problem. But if you are driving or in the middle of an important activity, it can have dramatic consequences.

Some of us acknowledge that we are addicted to caffeine and are willing to try to quit, at least temporarily. If this is your case, consider taking your time and easing your body into it. For example, if you are consuming three cups of coffee a day, start by decreasing it to one cup per day, rather than cutting yourself off completely. Otherwise, you might experience painful withdrawal symptoms such as headaches, mood swings, tiredness and sleepiness, and other flu-like symptoms. You can reduce the quantity little by little. If you drink mostly coffee, you can replace one cup of coffee with a cup of tea, which contains caffeine too, but less.

Find what works for you, and as always, be patient with yourself, acknowledge your efforts, and don't give up after the first failed attempt. Try to remember when you were trying to learn how to ride a bicycle: it didn't work the first time, but chances are you can ride today! Also, remember that we are not all affected by caffeine the same way. Some people are very sensitive and might not sleep when they have coffee after 10 am. Others might have coffee after dinner and sleep perfectly fine. Like everything else, we need to experiment to find the reason behind our poor sleep. If you are drinking coffee and experiencing issues with sleep, quitting coffee for a few weeks is an excellent place to start.

Alcohol

Don't skip this part, even if you drink only occasionally and very little!

Most people think of alcohol as having a depressant effect which can help them fall asleep. Though this is true, alcohol has other opposite effects that more than cancel out its relaxing aspect.

Now, you might feel like skipping this chapter because you are only having a glass of wine or a beer with dinner, and "that doesn't count as drinking". Research has established that even very low or moderate consumption of alcohol affects the quality of our sleep. Moderate consumption is one drink per day for women and up to two drinks per day for men, and low consumption is even less.

Anyone having issues with sleep should pay attention to their alcohol consumption, whether it comes from alcoholic drinks or medication that contains alcohol.

Alcohol can also disturb the sleep of people around us because it increases our risk of snoring and sleep apnea by making the muscles in our throat sag. This keeps the air from circulating as smoothly as it should. Alcohol consumption can also lead to haunting nightmares, which can put a damper on your restful sleep.

Alcohol, just like coffee or tea, has a diuretic effect: it makes you urinate more than usual. That makes it hard to get through the entire night without using the restroom. This is because alcohol acts on an antidiuretic hormone (ADH) called vasopressin. The role of vasopressin is to keep us from creating urine when we are at risk of getting dehydrated. Vasopressin maintains a healthy level of water in our body by keeping us from wanting to urinate. Alcohol decreases our levels of vasopressin and, as a result, increases the amount of urine we produce. No matter how dehydrated you get when drinking alcohol and no water, you will most likely still use the restroom because you won't have enough vasopressin produced to tell your body that it needs to hang on to the precious water.[16] This interruption might not be an issue for everyone, but for those who struggle to fall back asleep, it can be very problematic. Because alcohol is a strong diuretic, it will also dehydrate you, and you will most likely have to interrupt your sleep not just to go to the restroom but also later again to get a drink of water.

Finally, research has been done to measure the restfulness of a night using the subjects' heart rate variation. In other words, they measured the recovery aspect of sleep. For this study, they did not rely on perceptions or opinions from the participants. They directly measured their heart rate variation to establish how restful their sleep was. Researchers found that when they drank alcohol, their night was not as restful.[17] So even if you fall asleep quickly and maybe even sleep through the night, alcohol can cause you to feel poorly rested the next morning. Unfortunately, even a limited consumption of alcohol might have a deteriorating effect.

If you have a drink here and there and have sleep issues, it might be a good idea to stay off alcohol for at least a couple of weeks. Many people do a "dry month" in either October or January. I would encourage you to give it a try yourself and see if you notice any improvement in your sleep.

Cannabis

Because it helps with pain and with stress, we might think that cannabis helps with our sleep. Actually, it is not that straight forward. Cannabis has a negative influence on melatonin secretion, which can lead to our falling asleep later and later. According to a study by Deidre Conroy from the University of Michigan, 40% of people who smoked pot daily were struggling with insomnia, as opposed to only 10% of people who smoked occasionally.[18]

Once again, if sleep is a problem for you and you are using cannabis to relax and sleep better, you might want to look into your stressors and work on the root problems rather than trying to cope using external substances.

The Weight Factor

An Australian study revealed that the amount of cortisol our body releases after a meal is affected by our body weight.[19] According to this research, cortisol levels go up 51% after a meal in overweight participants. In comparison, they go up only 5% in non-overweight people. Cortisol, the stress hormone, is one of the most powerful enemies of sleep, and being overweight can make the issue worse if cortisol levels skyrocket after dinner or after a bedtime snack.[20]

PARASOMNIA

In medical terms, "para" means abnormal, and "somnia" means sleep. We describe parasomnia as something that goes wrong during someone's sleep. As opposed to insomnia, which keeps you from sleeping, parasomnia affects the quality of your sleep, the way you recover, and the way you feel when you wake up.

The list of parasomnias is long. Common ones are sleep apnea and restless legs syndrome, but there are also nightmares, night terrors, sleep-walking, sleep paralysis, teeth grinding, and many more. We will look primarily at sleep apnea, restless legs syndrome, and nightmares because they affect a more substantial part of the adult population I work with. It doesn't mean that other parasomnias cannot wreak havoc on your sleep, so if you sleep for a reasonable amount of time but wake up exhausted every morning, talk to a health care provider who might help you find out whether you are suffering from parasomnia.

Sleep Apnea

Sleep apnea happens when the air cannot go through our pharynx properly while we sleep. Most often, it is because of an obstruction of the pharynx – the cavity behind the nose and mouth – but sometimes (rarely), it is due to the nervous system not being able to maintain a regular breathing rhythm.

We will talk mostly about obstructions of the pharynx since it is the most common form of sleep apnea. The blockage can be complete or only partial. If it is complete, breathing stops for a short period. If it is partial, breathing does not stop, but the flow of oxygen is reduced.

Sleep apnea is a frequent issue in adults and is strongly linked to age and obesity. Men over 50, who are overweight and have a thick neck, are at higher risk of suffering from sleep apnea. Even more so if they drink alcohol, smoke, or take sleeping pills or tranquilizers. Women are not spared from sleep apnea, especially after they reach menopause.[21]

It is important to note the difference between sleep apnea and brief interruptions of our breathing rhythm that are common and normal. Sleep apnea usually becomes a problem when those interruptions last at least 10 seconds (with total interruption of the airflow) and happen very often throughout the night. When they happen five times per hour with symptoms such as daytime sleepiness and loud snoring, someone can be diagnosed as suffering from sleep apnea. When they happen 15 times per hour or more often, and without other symptoms, someone can still be diagnosed with sleep apnea.[22] When airflow is not completely blocked, we talk about sleep hypopnea instead of sleep apnea.

Again, it is important to remind ourselves that it is common to stop breathing a little here and there during the night. If it doesn't last long and doesn't happen often, it is just irregular breathing. But if you are not sure, seeking a diagnosis and advice from a health professional is essential.

The most common causes of sleep apnea are linked to the sagging of our pharynx muscles because they are too relaxed (due to age, medication, alcohol…) or because the pressure on them is too great (due to being overweight or obese). Too much pressure leads to much narrower airways.

Besides the fact that oxygen does not travel adequately through our system, sleep apnea is a problem because it leads to very poor-quality sleep. Every time our system notices that we are not getting a proper supply of air, it wakes us up to make sure we get back to regular breathing. We don't necessarily notice these interruptions in our sleep. However, they affect the quality of our nights because they keep us from spending the needed time in deep sleep and REM sleep, the two most restorative phases of sleep.

If you sleep with a partner, it might be easier to identify sleep apnea. Usually, after an episode of apnea, we gasp for air, and this can wake up the person next to us if they are in a period of light sleep. If sleep apnea episodes are frequent, chances are they will be noticed by the person who sleeps next to you.

If you sleep alone or your partner is a deep sleeper, you might not know that you have sleep apnea. Over time, though, you may experience symptoms during the day that show that you are not sleeping well through the night. If you are sleepy during the day or if you wake up tired despite sleeping well and long, then you might have sleep apnea.

The consequences of sleep apnea can be dangerous enough for you to take this problem seriously. If you ignore your sleep apnea, not only will you struggle to perform physically and intellectually, but you are also putting your health and life at risk. Sleep apnea, and the sleep deprivation that comes with it, put you at higher risk for depression, mood swings, headaches, and in the long run, diabetes, high blood pressure, and cardiovascular diseases, not to mention the dangers of dozing off while driving.

The tricky thing with sleep apnea is that its effects can worsen the apnea itself. Sleep apnea leads to low-quality sleep, which is directly linked to weight gain, lack of physical activity, and obesity. And since obesity can cause sleep apnea, the more weight we gain, the more prone to sleep apnea we are. Therefore, it is essential to see a doctor if you think you might suffer from sleep apnea.

If you are diagnosed with sleep apnea, you will be offered various solutions that you can discuss with your doctor. You can also work on improving things on your own, too. There are many steps you can take. One critical step is to change your lifestyle and make sure that your eating and drinking habits are not feeding your sleep apnea.

Drop the Booze

Alcohol at night is the first thing to eliminate from your life. Alcohol can make it increasingly difficult for you to sleep without interruptions, and you often wake up tired. Furthermore, alcohol leads to loss of muscle tone. Since sleep apnea mostly comes from the muscles of our pharynx sagging, alcohol exacerbates the problem.

Drop the Pills

Sedatives and tranquilizers can also worsen your apnea by overly relaxing the muscles in your body. This causes the pharynx to sag, and it narrows your airways. It could be beneficial to limit your intake of these kinds of medications. If you are having trouble sleeping and rely on sleeping pills to fall asleep, this might be a hard decision to make as your sleep quality might suffer in the short term. But it is worth considering such a long-term strategy to fix your sleep in a sustainable way. This is not a step to be taken lightly, though, so make sure you talk to your doctor first.

Drop the Weight

A healthy diet that allows you to manage your weight is also a natural way to reduce sleep apnea since the extra volume around your pharynx could cause an obstruction. Weight loss is not the most straightforward solution and might require several months or years of work. It is a long-term approach, but it shouldn't be dismissed if you are overweight and suffer from sleep apnea. Establishing a healthier lifestyle can definitely help, not only with sleep apnea but also with the quality of your sleep in general. I have seen so many clients come to me exhausted, without knowing why. After establishing a healthier lifestyle, with healthy eating and more physical activity, the quality of their sleep improved drastically, and their energy levels skyrocketed. This transformation is within reach when you take an approach that focuses on living a healthier life, rather than just losing weight.

Pick up the Ball

For many people, sleep apnea is mostly an issue when they sleep on their back. Sleeping on their side or their stomach can help the matter. To achieve this, a simple solution is to sew a pocket in the back of your pajamas and place a tennis ball in the pocket. Sleeping on your back will become uncomfortable enough for you to roll over and adopt a more apnea-proof position. This trick can also be used on your sleeping partner if they are snoring loudly and keeping you from sleeping well.

There are all kinds of mechanical devices that can reduce sleep apnea and snoring. We won't go into detail here, but from nose vents to smart pillows, you might find something that works for you. Ask your pharmacist or Google it!

It is essential to add that sleep apnea episodes, although they are influenced by all the factors listed above, can sometimes be due to someone's body shape. Again, it is important to get diagnosed and speak with a doctor about what is going on.

Restless Legs Syndrome

Restless Legs Syndrome (RLS) is also called Willis-Ekbom Disease. It is described by those who suffer from it as an uncomfortable sensation in the legs, most often the lower part of the leg. It can feel like burning, itching, throbbing, or even pins and needles. These symptoms often provoke an irresistible urge to move the legs or apply pressure on them. The feelings can go from mild discomfort to acute pain. The pain or discomfort from restless legs syndrome and the need to move around can often lead to poor quality sleep and, little by little, severe sleep deprivation.

Restless legs syndrome is a common issue and affects 7 to 10% of the population. Where sleep apnea is most often a problem for men, restless legs syndrome afflicts mostly women. Another difference between the sleep disorders is that as opposed to sleep apnea, which often starts as we get older, restless legs syndrome can begin at any age, even though symptoms are usually more frequent and last longer as we age.[23]

RLS affects sleep in two ways. Not only can it keep us awake purely and simply because the pain or discomfort keeps us from falling asleep but because the urge to move around keeps us from being in bed in the first place.

Once we are asleep, though, RLS can still affect the quality of our sleep. Even if we are not aware of it, moving around can lead to a lot of interruptions of our sleep during the night. These regular interruptions keep us from spending as much time as needed in deep sleep and thus keep us from recovering and feeling regenerated in the morning.

Some people are aware of their restless legs syndrome when it is time to fall asleep but don't realize that they also suffer from the condition during the night. Movements can be very subtle throughout the night, and you or a sleep partner might not notice them at all. What counts is not necessarily the scale of the movement but whether the movement slightly wakes you up and how frequently this happens throughout a night.

For this reason, if you know you suffer from restless legs syndrome and feel sleepy during the day, it is crucial to see a doctor who can set you up for a sleep analysis. Keep in mind how sleep deprivation can affect your health, your performance, and even be dangerous if you fall asleep while operating equipment or driving.

Restless Legs Syndrome, although frequent in the adult population, is still not very well understood, and it is unclear what might cause this sleep disorder. However, the following factors have been established as playing an essential role in RLS.

Parkinson's Disease

Insufficient dopamine seems to be largely involved in the development of restless legs syndrome, and since Parkinson's is directly linked to insufficient dopamine, Parkinson's might be the reason why certain people suffer from the syndrome.

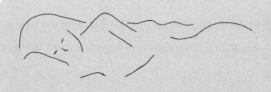

STORYTIME

A friend told me the story of Mary, who had been dealing with Restless Legs Syndrome for 20 years and had tried everything, including heavy-duty medication. One day, as she was desperately looking for answers in an online support group, Mary learned about rolling on a foam roller. Rolling her calves, hamstrings, and glutes for 12 to 15 minutes before bed to help relax her leg muscles allowed her to get off meds completely.

Mary discovered the foam roller seven years ago and has been using it successfully since. At times, she has to get up during the night and roll for a few extra minutes in order to relax her tight body parts. Afterward, she can fall back to sleep easily. She always keeps her foam roller available by her bed and has become used to this slight interruption during the night. The sleep she "loses" while rolling in the middle of the night is a small price to pay for being able to enjoy good-quality sleep the rest of the night.

Iron Deficiency

An iron deficiency might also be the reason you suffer from RLS. It is easy to check your iron levels: a simple blood test might help you discover whether you are iron deficient, though not necessarily anemic. In such instances, taking iron supplements prescribed by your physician could be enough to take care of your syndrome.

Medical Conditions

Conditions such as diabetes or kidney failure might also lead to the development of restless legs syndrome. Just as for Parkinson's and iron deficiency, treating the medical condition will usually allow for symptoms of restless legs syndrome to disappear or at least drastically diminish.

Pregnancy

The last trimester of pregnancy has been linked to increased occurrences of restless legs syndrome. Often, symptoms disappear after the pregnancy is over, but not always. Think about when the symptoms of RLS started bothering you.

Medication

Certain antipsychotics and antidepressants, as well as some cold and allergy medicines, can either be the source of RLS or can increase the symptoms when the problem is already present. If you are taking medication and experiencing RLS, check side effects with your healthcare provider.

Lifestyle

Alcohol, chocolate, tea, tobacco, coffee, and caffeine-containing foods and drinks can either induce RLS or worsen its symptoms. In addition, sleep deprivation can also lead to RLS.

Sometimes, Restless Legs Syndrome cannot be linked back to any condition, lifestyle habit, or temporary state such as pregnancy. RLS can be passed down hereditarily, and in this case, it is a much more difficult problem to tackle.

If you suffer from Restless Legs Syndrome, the first step, after following the recommendations of your healthcare provider, is to track your sleep quality, as well as your food and liquid intake. This will allow you to spot habits and behaviors that might be reasons for the problem. If you notice that your lifestyle is far from optimal when it comes to RLS, it is essential to take measures to resolve this while still tracking your sleep quality. Ideally, you will zero in on one lifestyle change at a time to keep from getting overwhelmed. Don't expect improvement within days or even weeks. It might take a few months for a lifestyle change to affect the quality of your sleep, so be consistent and give it some time. I will walk you through the whole process step by step in the next chapter, so don't worry, you are not alone in this.

If lifestyle is not the problem and you have implemented all the changes necessary without success, consider seeing a doctor so that other causes can be ruled out. Establishing a healthier lifestyle might allow you to reduce your intake of certain medications, but if you are taking medicine that you believe might be the reason for your RLS, I would also recommend talking to your doctor about finding an alternative medication.

Nightmares

Adult nightmares are sometimes tricky to handle. They can wake us up regularly and make it scary or difficult to go back to sleep. They can be so terrifying that we don't want to sleep in the first place. Nightmares might keep us from turning off the lights, which disturbs our melatonin production, and they can create a feeling of insecurity that keeps us from relaxing and prevents our brain waves from slowing down.

If we don't have nightmares, maybe our partner's nightmares are an issue, especially if they are acting out while dreaming, which can be extremely disrupting and also scary or even dangerous. If your other half is acting out their nightmares regularly after a certain age (50 or 60), ask them to see a doctor because this can be an early symptom of Parkinson's Disease. Since there are treatments available, getting things checked out early is best.

It is essential to know that alcohol has a nightmare-promoting effect, and so do antidepressants and anti-anxiety medication. Reducing alcohol around dinner time can have a positive impact on your sleep in many ways. And talking to your health care provider about nightmares might lead to beneficial tweaks in your medication regimen.

• • •

By now, you probably have a few ideas of why your sleep might be broken. Take a few minutes and write down below the reasons why you think you don't sleep well:

_____

_____

_____

_____

With everything you have learned already, chances are you also have an idea of a few steps you could already take to improve your sleep. If that's the case, don't wait! If you have identified obvious reasons for your broken sleep, then you can start experimenting with changes immediately, even before designing your very own winning sleep plan.

I recommend writing below the changes you want to experiment with right away. It will give you a place to start.

Obvious changes I will experiment with right away:

_____

_____

_____

_____

_____

If you are not inspired yet, no problem. We will get to it in the next chapter. But first, it is essential to pause for a minute and acknowledge the steps you have already taken if you have followed the process of this book so far.

By now, you have completed the AWARENESS PHASE.

You learned how sleep works and why it is vital for good health and wellness. You also gained a better understanding of the most common reasons why so many of us struggle with sleep and you discovered the five keys to sleeping well:

- Enough time for sleep
- Enough tiredness
- Harmony with your internal clock
- Melatonin release
- Slower brain waves

Then, you took the time to observe your sleep patterns and should know a lot more about what your current sleep looks like, what your natural needs are, and what you can aim for when you want to improve your sleep. If you have not gathered that data yet, don't worry, it is not too late. Do the work now and find out:

- Whether or not you are sleep-deprived (Sleep Quiz, chapter two);
- How much time you dedicate to sleep each night (Sleep Tracker, chapter two);
- How much time you ACTUALLY sleep each night (Sleep Tracker, chapter two);
- When you need to sleep (Chronotype Spotter or Vacation Experiment, chapter three);
- How long you need to sleep (Chronotype Spotter, or Vacation Experiment, or Incremental Method, chapter three)

You can keep track of what you have done and what's left to do by checking off the steps below.

LEARN

□ **Hidden Powers of Sleep**
Chapter 1

□ **Your Starting Point**
Sleep Quiz, Sleep Tracker
Chapter 2

□ **Mechanics of Sleep**
Chapter 3

□ **Your Sleep Needs**
Chronotype Spotter, or Vacation Experiment, or Incremental Method
Chapter 3

□ **Five Keys to Sleeping Well**
Chapter 4

□ **Common Reasons for Poor Sleep**
Chapter 5

©2021 Stella Loichot

Knowledge is power.

With everything you have learned so far about yourself and about sleep, it is now time to create a winning sleep plan that fits your lifestyle and allows you to finally reach your goals.

Let's get into ACTION!

PART II
Action

"Imperfect action is better than perfect inaction."
~Harry Truman, maybe...

This quote might or might not be from Harry Truman. What is certain, though, is that I heard it for the first time from Kathleen Legrys, my business mentor, and have been trying my best to abide by it every single day since. It has propelled me forward.

In this second part of the book, you will design and implement your winning sleep plan step by step. To help you with that, I will provide 25 real-life situations addressing the most common problems, and we will review a few special cases such as night shift, menopause, and parenting.

But before you dive headfirst into designing your winning sleep plan, I want to remind you that some people don't fit the mold. A small percentage of us need less sleep than the general population. We have mentioned earlier that the recommendation for most healthy adults is to sleep seven to nine hours per night and seven to eight hours for older adults. Still, if you don't sleep that long and yet feel alert and full of energy during the day without unconsciously relying on crutches such as coffee, soda, snacks, and high levels of stress, the chances are that there is no problem with your sleep. You may just belong to the very few people who need little sleep.

By the same token, if you wake up systematically in the middle of the night, it is crucial to figure out whether it is a natural tendency or an actual sleep disruption. If you wake up every single night at approximately the same time and still feel refreshed and ready to thrive in the morning without relying on caffeine or other external help, you can embrace the fact that your body wants to be active at a specific time every night. It might not be a sleep issue.

If it doesn't stress you out too much (and as a result won't lead to frustration and maybe insomnia), you can use that extra time to do something that won't get your brain too active. No screen, obviously. You can read, sort some laundry, write in a gratitude journal, or cut veggies for the next day. I personally enjoy writing letters and sending cards to relatives in France. It is essential to pick an activity that's not challenging intellectually, not too exciting or frustrating, and to make sure it is not something you would start looking forward to doing each night when you go to bed. Otherwise, you might start waking up every night in anticipation of that activity.

Don't waste your time trying to fit into the "sleep-through-the-night" mold if you don't belong there. Use your time wisely; make sure that what you do won't keep you from falling back asleep as you would usually if you stayed in bed.

Now, if your sleep needs fixing, here is the process that will help you build your unique sleep improvement plan.

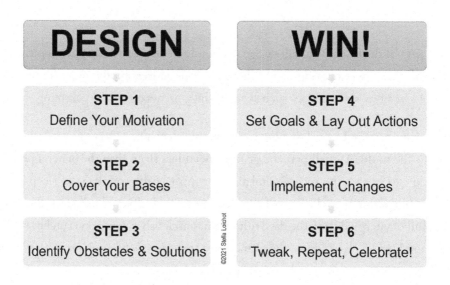

Are you ready to design your winning sleep plan? Let's go!

CHAPTER SIX
Your Winning Sleep Plan

STEP ONE: BUILD MOTIVATION

Reasons for Better Sleep

I personally could not maintain my efforts if I didn't observe, daily, the direct effect of chronic sleep deprivation on my weight and mood. Your motivators differ from mine and those of others around you. You might be more concerned about intellectual performance or a more youthful-looking skin and diminished bags under the eyes, while your neighbor might be in it for athletic performance or the fear of memory loss.

No matter what gets you to work on your sleep, it is crucial that you write a list of all the things that will change in your life if you improve your sleep. You can also write down all the things that will deteriorate if you do not adjust your sleep. Ideally, you have the two lists next to each other for an even more powerful motivator.

Use the Reasons for Better Sleep worksheet to list everything that will change in your life once you sleep better. Try to be as specific as possible. The longer the list, the easier it will be for you to do the work later on. You can access the Reasons for Better Sleep worksheet at allonZcoaching.com/sleepitoff with the password SLEEP_IT_OFF.

To get you inspired, there are a few examples on the following page.

Reasons for Better Sleep

Example

If I improve my sleep...	If I don't do anything...
Won't feel as hungry all day	Won't lose weight
Easier life (no fatigue)	Blood pressure will rise
Less snacking: weight loss	I will get diabetes
I won't drink as much coffee	I will keep thinking about my weight all the time
Save money on snacks/coffee	Relationship with food will get even worse
More productive mornings	Will age faster
Less tired after work: will run	Won't keep up with grandkids
More sex drive, better relationship	More lines; skin and face will look older
No more bags under my eyes	
...	

Reasons for Better Sleep

Download online

Find as many reasons to improve your sleep as possible.
The longer the list, the easier it will be to stay motivated.

If I improve my sleep...	If I don't do anything...

Define Your WHY

There might be times when you lose your focus, feel discouraged, and want to give up because it is a long process and rewards might not be instant. For that reason, it is essential to know exactly, deep down, why you want to improve your sleep. You cannot settle for the very first answer that crosses your mind because it is your profound motivation that will keep you going when you want to quit.

After I collapsed in 2014 and decided to bring sleep back into my life, I had to make room in my schedule for three extra hours of sleep. You can imagine the challenge since nothing else had changed in my life, except that I was not participating in triathlon races anymore. At first, I completely stopped exercising, so that gave me quite a lot of free time, but soon enough, I went back to being physically active and the time crush became real. It might have been easier if I had enjoyed sleeping in the first place. But that's not the case, and you know that by now: lying unconscious in my bed falls low for me on the enjoyment scale. As a result, I need to have a powerful motivation to stay dedicated to reaching my sleep goals. One of my many motivators for sleeping more is that it is the only way to keep my weight under control. As soon as I get sleep-deprived, extra pounds pile up. If my "why" is simply to maintain my weight, here is what will happen. I will be disciplined for a few weeks and will make time for sleep. I might purchase blackout curtains, turn off my phone, and not drink wine with dinner. I will take lots of steps that will be uncomfortable and inconvenient. If they were not, I would have taken those steps years ago. And then one day, I won't be able to go to bed as planned because of work, a book to write, or the cat throwing up on the carpet. Then my husband will prepare a nice meal and bring out the wine. Everyday challenges will come back full blast into my life, and either I will stop noticing them and lose my focus, or I will make the conscious decision that this whole thing is too hard and a few extra pounds are not worth the battle. I will easily convince myself that this is not worth it and will happily go back to chronic sleep deprivation until I hit the wall again.

Now, because I worked hard on defining a more profound reason why it is essential for me to maintain my weight, things have turned out differently. Here was my thought process: "I want to keep my weight under control *because* I want to show food lovers like me that it is possible to stay at a healthy weight even if we love cheese, bread, and chocolate. It is possible to become healthy, even if we have been overweight and battled with yo-yo dieting for many years. It is possible to enjoy life even if we have a sweet tooth. I want to inspire those who have struggled with food and cravings their entire life *because* I want to give them hope, even if they believe that they will never manage their weight since they have tried every single diet out there already. **Giving hope and guiding others to success is my mission**. It is the reason I created my own practice as a health and wellness coach. My work relies on setting an example, and if I can't make it happen in my own life, then I feel that I am lying to myself and lying to all those I work with. That's why I have to protect my sleep and maintain my health and my weight. Otherwise, I lose track of my mission and I don't feel true to myself. That's one of the profound reasons why sleep is so important to me. When I want to cut my sleep short, this is what I remind myself of.

If I define my WHY this way, when life gets tricky and keeps me from making progress in my journey, I might still lapse and sleep poorly for a while, but I won't lose sight of my goal, and I will get back on track because I need to stay true to my purpose. I won't give up, because it is not just about a few pounds anymore; it is way bigger than that.

This is only one example. I could also have defined my WHY around my being a role model for my children and thus feeling confident as a mom. We often have several WHYs. You can explore them all, or you can choose one. Just make sure, once again, that you are going deep under the surface because you need something strong to carry you along the journey.

To define your profound WHY, answer all the questions on the Define Your Why worksheet. Make sure you go all the way through the process. Don't stop after answering the first "why?" even if you are tempted to do so. Keep digging.

Define Your Why

Example

START HERE! I want to sleep better because...

↓

Being tired puts me in a bad mood

It's important because... →

Want to be less irritable with kids

Important because...

Write your profound WHY here:

When I sleep well and am rested, I can handle both my family and my job and that makes me feel like I am successful at life. That feeling gives me energy and power!

Important because...

Feel like a bad mom. Feel guilty to love my career so much

← important to me because...

I feel bad when I am not patient with kids

Define Your Why

Download online

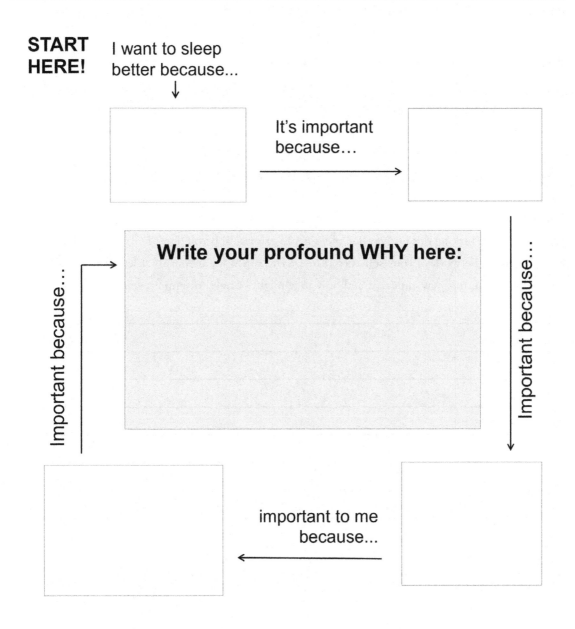

START HERE!

I want to sleep better because...

It's important because...

Write your profound WHY here:

Important because...

Important because...

important to me because...

STEP TWO: COVER YOUR BASES

Covering your bases before you work on the specifics of your situation allows you to experience some benefits right away. We are all unique, yes. And that's why you need to create your own plan if you want to reach your goals. But we are also all human and have a lot in common. By implementing the following basic changes, you could most likely hit the mark on many personal issues.

Make Sleep Your Priority and Go Public

The very first step that we should all take to sleep well and enough is to make sure we are putting sleep at or near the top of our priority list. Others might not be doing the same, and may not understand, as our world is ravaged by sleep deprivation. Chances are many people around you do not value sleep as much as they should, so your decision to commit to improving your sleep will either seem unimportant to them or might even bother them.

I highly recommend that you tell people around you that you are working on improving your sleep and that you are making this project one of your top priorities. If you don't feel comfortable informing your entire network of your self-care plans, write down the names of at least three people you will talk to about this new endeavor and how they might be able to support you.

_____

_____

_____

_____

_____

_____

_____

_____

_____

_____

_____

_____

_____

"Going public" ensures that everybody around you knows what you are trying to achieve and understands why you are making the changes you are making – and why you might be grumpy once you quit coffee. To go a step further, it is an excellent idea to explain to surrounding people the benefits that they might get from helping you improve your sleep. If they realize that when you sleep more, you are more patient, you have more energy to do things with them or for them, and you are happier and bring more to the world, they might not be as frustrated. They might even try to encourage you, support you, and keep you accountable if you tell them how they can be your ally. This would be of tremendous help.

To map out in more detail how you can engage the people around you, use the Support System worksheet from your workbook and make sure you act on it.

Eat Healthily and Regularly

When working with clients on weight loss, it is thrilling to see the transformation they experience in their sleeping patterns after only a few weeks of adopting a healthier diet.

If you are not doing this yet, start right here before you move on to the next phase of exploring each specific solution that might work for you.

Incorporate more whole foods into your diet, especially more fiber from vegetables, fruits, and non-processed grains and beans. Eat less processed food and fast food, and try to eat less fried food and fatty meat, especially at dinner. Replacing saturated animal fat with healthy plant-based fat has a tremendous impact on sleep quality.

 DID YOU KNOW?

One thing that surprised me when I moved to the United States 20 years ago was the cultural differences related to the timing of meals. I didn't notice at first, but the first time I went back to France to visit family, it became apparent. Every time I wanted to plan a hike, a stroll in town, or a visit to a friend, I had to make sure it would not interfere with a meal. In France, mealtimes are, to a certain extent, set in stone. The French schedule their activities and work meetings around their meals. In the United States, we schedule our activities in a way that allows us to fit as much as possible into a day, and we grab food whenever there is an opportunity. Our meals have to fit into our busy lives, and if there is no room for lunch, we just skip it and snack later. In France, activities have to fit in around the meals, not the other way around. It might not seem like such an enormous difference, but it has serious consequences not only on food intake but also on stress, relationships, and sleep. There is no good or bad, but it is essential to keep in mind that our habits are very cultural and that we can change them more than we think if we stop and reflect on them.

Try to have regular meals throughout the day rather than snacking or eating whenever your busy life allows for it, and make sure that your days are structured in a way that doesn't leave too much room for snacking. Eating your meals around the same time every day can give your body a sense of routine, and it will be even more beneficial if you finish dinner at least two hours before going to bed.

It is essential to know that about 90% of the serotonin we produce is made in our guts. If you remember, serotonin is the precursor to the sleep hormone melatonin. Making sure that you eat a diet rich in whole foods, fiber, and probiotics can help you take care of your digestive tract and maintain its activity and hormone production level where it should be.[1] Relatively recent research has shown that "Total microbiome diversity was positively correlated with increased sleep efficiency and total sleep time, and was negatively correlated with wake after sleep onset".[2] This means that the more variety you have in your diet – assuming that it is a healthy diet rich in plants and whole foods – the better you could sleep.

To produce serotonin, our guts need tryptophan. Tryptophan is an amino acid present in such foods as poultry, shellfish, meat, peanuts, almonds, pumpkin seeds, and soy, and it also helps boost melatonin production.[3] This is another excellent example of why having a varied diet and eating healthy whole foods are so essential for our health. If we eliminate an entire food group for a restrictive diet, we might experience some surprising side effects, such as poor sleep.

Just by reducing highly processed foods and increasing whole foods in your daily eating, chances are you will notice a difference in your sleep.

Eat Less

This recommendation might not apply to you, and maybe you already have your food intake dialed in. If that is the case, just move on. Yet if you are overweight and struggling with sleep, and especially if you tend to wake up in the middle of the night hot, agitated, and thirsty, chances are that your daily energy intake exceeds your energy expenditure. This means that you eat more calories during the day than you burn through physical activity. We have already mentioned the fact that overeating at dinnertime might hinder your sleep. But it is not just about dinner and late-night snacks. Making sure you eat a reasonable number of calories throughout the day is an important step. One way to do so is to stop eating once you feel 80% full, rather than eat until you feel completely satiated. You can also use smaller dinner plates and avoid going for seconds. Preparing smaller quantities of food works wonders too, or cooking more but freezing extra portions right away for a future meal.

There are many other ways to control the size of your portions. This topic will be covered in detail in another book.

Move More

If you also direct your attention to being more active throughout the day and spending more time outside, you will most likely start sleeping better and longer and feel more invigorated in the morning when you wake up. According to the U.S. Department of Health and Human Services, not even 5% of American adults perform the 30 minutes of daily physical activity that are recommended for good health.[4] Things look grim globally too, with more than 80% of adolescents in the world not being active enough.[5] Just like eating less, moving more is an excellent step to take even before you figure out what the reasons might be for your lack of sleep. It also helps you along your weight loss journey, and if you are at risk for type 2 diabetes, you can enjoy great benefits from being more physically active.

Listen to Your Body

Try to align your sleep routine with your biological clock rather than adjusting it to the people around you. At the same time, get your body used to having a regular schedule, not only at night but also during the day.

To listen to your body, you need to get rid of all the noise that is covering up the cues your body is trying to send you. You may need to reduce caffeine, alcohol, and cannabis dramatically, and you need to be as honest with yourself as you can. If you play the victim and blame your lack of sleep on everything and everyone, it might make you feel a bit better but it won't help you solve the problem. It is critical that you look at your lifestyle the way an outsider would, without blame, without judgment, but also without trying to find excuses. Take charge, take responsibility, and try to observe, objectively and with self-compassion, how your body reacts to the way you are treating it.

STEP THREE: IDENTIFY ISSUES AND SOLUTIONS

What Keeps You from Sleeping

If you want to be successful, you need to know what the unique factors are that keep you from sleeping well. Having that knowledge is the only way you can take impactful actions. Otherwise, you will waste your efforts and energy on changes that won't make a difference.

Knowing everything you know now, you might already have a few ideas as to what the issues are. If you do, start writing a list. Be as specific as possible. It could look like this:

- Hard to unwind at night, worried about work
- Not enough tiredness accumulated (nap, sitting all day)
- Not enough time to sleep (has never been a priority)
- Eat too late at night, close to bedtime
- A glass of white wine after coming home from work
- Screen time after dinner
- Go to bed too late

Use the Obstacles & Solutions worksheet to list as many obstacles to good sleep you can think of in the left column. Of course, this worksheet is alsoin your workbook if you have printed it. Don't think about solutions, yet. Try to identify as many problems as possible so that your list is long.

In case you need additional help with that task, I have created for you a BONUS Checklist with 100 Common Sleep-Killers. You can download it at allonZcoaching.com/sleepitoff for extra support. It will help you get started if you don't know what might contribute to your lack of sleep.

Potential Solutions

Now that you have identified many reasons for your sleep struggles, it is time to brainstorm a few ways you could eliminate them or diminish their impact. Write them all down on the Obstacles & Solutions worksheet.

Don't worry if you can't find ideas to mitigate all the problems, but do your best to find as many as possible, and even several action steps for each issue. Brainstorming with someone else can be an excellent idea. Sometimes, we are so caught up in our own lives and habits that we don't even realize that there might be another way to do things.

If, deep inside, you feel that there is nothing you can do about your sleep problems, then the first step in your solution should be to self-reflect on why you think this way and decide whether right now is a good time for you to start your sleep improvement journey.

Obstacles & Solutions

Example

Existing Obstacles	Potential Solutions
Cat chewing dry food at 5 am	Cat food downstairs White noise app to cover chewing
Worried I won't hear alarm	Teach kids how to use alarm Ask Joe to call from work at 8
Tired at 9 but in bed at 11 pm	Go to bed 15 minutes earlier until I get to 9 pm
Night time routine with kids is too long	Brainstorm ideas with Joe Take turn with Joe?
Hard to wind down, so much to do!	Meditation, turn off screen after dinner, stretching, walk, brain dump, write to-do list before bed
Joe's snoring	Sleep in guest room for a while

Obstacles & Solutions

Download online

This list is an evolving document!
Add to both columns as you learn more about yourself
and experiment with solutions.

Existing Obstacles	Potential Solutions

If you don't feel ready or able to work on your sleep just yet and to invest the required time and energy to be successful, don't beat yourself up. There are times when we have so much to juggle that we don't have the spare capacity to take on the extra responsibility that comes with knowledge and power, even if our goal is to be healthier and happier. If that's where you are, please don't judge yourself. Keep learning, keep being open, and eventually, you will feel ready to take care of yourself and start changing your lifestyle. Not being ready to take charge doesn't make you a lesser person. It only means that you might need a little more time, maybe a stronger motivation, or perhaps some extra support.

7-Day Journaling

Identifying obstacles and solutions off the top of your head is a good place to start. But if you are serious about changing your lifestyle, you need to go a step further. This is where detailed tracking of your daily routine – everything you do, eat, drink, and feel for a couple of weeks – can be extremely helpful. Use the Daily Journal and fill it out every single day for at least seven days. This will allow you to identify many more issues in your current way of life, and you will end up with a much longer list of obstacles and potential solutions. You can print as many Daily Journal pages as you want to from the downloadable companion workbook.

If you track thoughtfully and are very intentional about this work, your list of improvement ideas will grow quickly and you will discover that you truly have the power to change your life and improve your sleep. It can be challenging to identify sleep-damaging behaviors on your own; if that is the case, working with a behavioral change specialist might be necessary.

When you track, it is crucial to be very detailed about the way you feel. Waking up in the morning with puffy eyes or a cloudy brain, sweating heavily or having cramps at night, suffering from acid reflux or headaches during the day are all things that you should record. Everything that you notice should find its place in your tracking log, whether it is bad breath, bloating, white tongue, irritability, or cravings. The more detailed your journal is, the easier it will be to identify culprits of your poor sleep. Write everything down as you go through your day. Don't wait until the end of the day to remember, because it won't be an accurate recollection. Keeping your journal with you at all times for a week or two is a minor price to pay considering the fantastic value you can get out of this exercise. If you find it too cumbersome, you can also take very detailed notes throughout the day in a small notebook and copy everything into your Daily Journal at the end of the day.

It is now time to track your daily food intake, activities, and feelings for seven days.

Daily Journal

Example

TIME	Wake up (with/without alarm, sleep quality, how do you feel?)
6:40	Alarm, tired, could sleep 2 more hours

TIME	Food/Beverage & Physical Activity	How do you feel?
7 am	Breakfast: scrambled eggs + fruit salad + bagel + butter + coffee	Sleepy, better after
12 pm	Walked to sushi place	Glad I didn't drive
12:30 pm	Lunch: sushi + leftover chicken noodle soup + 2 chocolate cookies	Sleepy 1 hour after lunch
7 pm	Dinner: Chicken alfredo pasta + 1 red wine + 5 girl scout cookies	Full after seconds, but still wanted cookies
10 pm	Finished box of cookies	Frustrated

Stress (trigger, level, duration...)
Fight with Mike, ruined my night as I was ruminating after the call

What are you doing during the 2 hours before bedtime?
Called Mike (mistake!) + took a bath (relaxing!) + TV + ate cookies

Time you go to bed and stop ALL activities: 10:30 pm
How are you feeling? Frustrated by phone call, mad about the cookies

NOTES: Phone calls with Mike are rarely smooth. I could call him around lunch time. I sat almost all day.

Daily Journal

Download online

TIME	Wake up (with/without alarm, sleep quality, how do you feel?)	

TIME	Food/Beverage & Physical Activity	How do you feel?

Stress (trigger, level, duration...)

What are you doing during the 2 hours before bedtime?

Time you go to bed and stop ALL activities:
How are you feeling?

NOTES:

Identify Positive Habits

It is important to be aware of all the sleep-promoting habits you already have. This shows you that you are already doing good work, which can be very motivational. Make sure you don't forget about these positive habits or behaviors and don't lose them along the way while you work on changing your harmful practices. Identifying them might also help you reinforce them.

Once you have logged in your journal for one or two weeks, the first step of your action plan is to list all the things you do that are helping you sleep. For example, maybe you wake up every single day at the same time, or perhaps you walk to and from work every day. Maybe your room is quiet and cool, and you don't let anyone in at night who could disturb you. These are examples of positive actions that will benefit your sleep.

Look at your Daily Journal, day by day, and list your sleep-promoting behaviors. They need to be protected throughout your journey, and some of them can even be amplified.

List your sleep-promoting habits below and decide which ones you could intensify and how. Of course, you can also write your list of sleep-promoting habits in the Sleep-Promoting Habits worksheet in your printed workbook.

_____

_____

_____

_____

_____

_____

_____

_____

_____

_____

_____

_____

Pinpoint Harmful Behaviors and Environment

After identifying all your sleep-promoting habits, the next step is to write a (long) list of all the reasons you might not sleep well: pets waking you up, worries (be specific), noises (describe them), lack of time, coffee, alcohol, heavy meals, pain, etc. You started this list earlier when you filled out the Obstacles & Solutions worksheet. It is now time to use the data collected in your Daily Journal, to add many more ideas to that list.

Look at everything you have reported in your Daily Journal and, using the knowledge you have gained in the first part of this book, find out what needs to be changed. Don't limit yourself to what you believe you can change. Write everything that is not actively helping you sleep, even if you can't do anything about it right now.

For even more ideas, you can also use the Sleep Tracker that you filled out in chapter two and the Chronotype Spotter from chapter three. You have gathered a lot of data about yourself and your lifestyle. Now is the time to use it and analyze it. If you find it hard to see how your lifestyle might keep you from sleeping well, don't assume that there is nothing you can do. Reach out to someone who will help you identify potential issues. A coach is a great option, obviously, but sometimes, even a friend can help you see what is right in front of you. Remember, the more reasons for not sleeping you come up with, the more power you will have to improve your sleep.

Don't worry if your list is short. Focusing on changes that seem the most obvious to you is a perfect way to get started and move in the right direction. You can always look for more improvement points later on, so consider this list an evolving resource. You will keep adding potential issues and solutions as you go.

Don't worry, either, if the list is long and daunting. Just write everything that might be an issue and you will prioritize in the next step. You might not have to work through the entire list before you improve your sleep significantly.

Before you start implementing changes, you can make sure that you have everything you need to succeed, using the checklist on the following page.

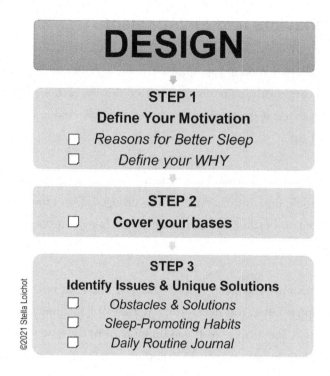

You have done all the work – it is now time to WIN! This is the home run and the most rewarding phase of your plan. It looks like this:

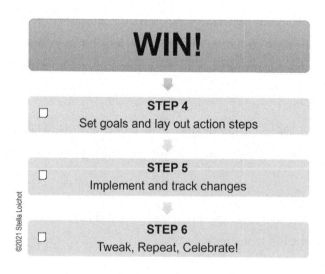

STEP FOUR: SET GOALS AND LAY OUT ACTION STEPS

Decide what you want to achieve within two or three months, and what you will do, concretely, to get there. Write the result you are aiming for at the top of your Winning Sleep Plan Tracker (see worksheet on page 120). Don't skip this phase, or you will lose track of what you are trying to achieve, and also, you won't be able to acknowledge the progress you make.

Be as specific as possible when you write what your goal is. For example, a goal could be: "sleep at least seven hours every night," or "wake up only once per night," or "wake up fully rested four times per week." Keep your goal or goals specific and detailed. If your goal is to "sleep well," how will you know you have reached it? Once your sleep improves, you will most likely want to sleep even better and will forget how miserable your sleep was before. Furthermore, if you work hard to sleep better but don't know if your efforts are paying off, you will want to give up. Your goals have to be specific and measurable if you want them to motivate you and allow you to see progress.

Make sure you don't start with a goal that you can't reach within two or three months. It is ok to have big goals, but you'll have more success by breaking your big goal into small steps.

If you have been waking up five times per night for the past three years, your goal could be to wake up only twice per night. This would be a significant improvement and might happen within a few weeks. Once you reach that goal, you can move on to the next step. Even though sleeping through the night might be your ultimate goal, aim for something more realistic at first. Setting goals that you can achieve within eight to twelve weeks, rather than very long-term goals, can help you stay focused and motivated. They also make the entire process more exciting and flexible, as you can reassess more frequently and revise your objectives downwards if needed without a crippling sense of failure.

 DID YOU KNOW?

It might surprise you to hear that, as a health coach and behavioral change specialist, I often support my clients by slowing them down and encouraging them to set smaller and more achievable goals. My role is not to be their cheerleader but the pacer who will curb their enthusiasm to make sure they can run the distance. A recurring cause of failure we encounter, no matter what the endeavor, is setting the bar too high and getting discouraged when we can't live up to our expectations or those of others. It is imperative to keep in mind that our goals are just the stepping stones to a result. If you ever learned how to drive a car, you know that your first step was not to hit the freeway. And yet, you knew from the very beginning that you would eventually get there. You most likely started in a parking lot, and gradually made it to busy streets and highways. Starting small is the key to success; don't see it as a lack of ambition.

Once you have clarified your goal for the two or three months to come, it is time to define the first action steps that will help you reach it. As you do so, make sure you do not overwhelm yourself with too many action steps at once. Use the Obstacles & Solutions worksheet that you already filled out. From that worksheet, pick a couple of solutions (aka action steps) that you could experiment with as soon as possible. Write these steps on the Winning Sleep Plan Tracker that is in your workbook, and keep track of what you are doing.

Again, don't cover every sleep issue and every potential solution right away. You need to start somewhere, and there is no rush and no reason to overwhelm yourself with too many things to focus on.

If you feel at a loss, here are a few extra examples for your action plan.

Example #1

GOAL: Sleep two hours longer each weeknight

Timeframe: three months

ACTION STEPS for the coming week:

- Go to bed 20 minutes earlier
- Stop snoozing: sleep 10 minutes longer
- Set the alarm far away from the bed so that I have to get up to turn it off

Example #2

GOAL: Reduce stress level two nights per week

Timeframe: three months

ACTION STEPS for the coming week:

- No computer or phone after dinner – Can't check emails
- Gentle 30-minute walk after dinner
- Easy-to-read book to take my mind away from daily worries

Your goal doesn't have to be directly sleep-related. Since you now understand all the requirements that need to be met for you to sleep better, you can also set a goal that is directly linked to your lifestyle. This is your action plan. Make sure it seems achievable and that it applies to you and your daily routine.

Winning Sleep Plan Tracker

Example

My goal for the coming __2__ months is: fall asleep 1 hour earlier than what I am used to

This week, I will experiment with the steps below and track my progress.

Action Step / New Habit	Day 1	Day 2	Day 3	Day 4	Day 5	Day 6	Day 7
Dinner 6 instead of 7pm	X	X			X	X	
No screen after dinner	X		X				X
30-minute night walk	X		X	X	X	X	X

Notes: Night walk is very enjoyable. Need to put phone away, otherwise can't resist. I slept better when I didn't have meat for dinner. Will focus on that next week.

Winning Sleep Plan Tracker

Download online

My goal for the coming _____ months is: _____

_____

This week, I will experiment with the steps below and track my progress.

Action Step / New Habit	Day 1	Day 2	Day 3	Day 4	Day 5	Day 6	Day 7

Notes: _____

_____

_____

Example #3

GOAL: Walk 10,000 steps daily

Timeframe: two months

ACTION STEPS for the coming week:

- Get off bus two stops early on weekdays
- Take 30-minute walk on Saturday and Sunday morning

Example #4

GOAL: Reduce meat intake by 20%

Timeframe: 2 months

ACTION STEPS for the coming week:

- Eat fish or seafood two times per week for dinner
- Eat hummus with celery sticks instead of salami for snacks

Your action steps need to be very specific. If you commit to "eating a healthy dinner" or "walking more," this is not specific enough. You won't know when you have achieved these steps. If you are not sure how specific your action steps should be, imagine that someone is observing everything you do, but they have no clue about where you are starting from and what your end goal is. Will they be able to evaluate your achievements? They might not know what a "healthy dinner" is. But they will be able to assess if half of your plate is covered with vegetables and they will easily count how many glasses of wine you have for dinner. They might not know what "walking more" means exactly, but they will know whether you have walked 5 or 45 minutes.

It is also critical that your action steps be relatively easy to implement. You are not trying to bring about a revolution into your daily routine. At least, not within a couple of weeks. Your actions will eventually turn your life upside down (downside up, actually!), but this will happen gradually, as you stack up new sleep-promoting habits.

Here is a simple way to test whether an action step is reachable. Ask yourself two questions:

- Am I at least 80% sure that I will do this?
- Will I be able to do this at least 80% of the time?

If the answer is yes to at least one of these questions, your action step is most likely within reach. Otherwise, you will want to step it down a little. This method was inspired by Christine Suter, a Professional Life Coach I deeply trust and respect.[6] You can use it in all areas of your life.

Focus on areas of life where you have the most power and also on action steps that will have the most impact. Find a balance between small changes that are easy to implement and more significant and influential modifications that might take more time and effort. Don't direct your attention to things over which you don't have control. If your street is loud and busy, you won't be able to change that, but you might get some relief using earplugs or white noise in your bedroom. If your partner snores loudly despite all their efforts, getting mad at them won't make a difference, but you might consider sleeping somewhere else if at all possible. Not everybody has a spare room, of course, or even a couch, but try to concentrate on your goal and forget society's standards. If sleeping on a mat in the kitchen means that you will be more rested the next day, it is worth trying. Sleeping well sometimes requires that you make tough choices, and you are the only one able to decide which sacrifices are worth it and which are not. Just keep in mind that you won't improve your sleep if you don't implement some changes.

STEP FIVE: IMPLEMENT CHANGES

Now that you have a written plan, know what you want to achieve, and have defined action steps you can take, it is time to implement your plan and experiment with your action steps.

Add a checkmark every time you successfully take the step you were planning on taking. Don't worry if you skip one day here and there. It is not about perfection; it is all about consistency in the long term. Be kind to yourself, while also making sure to stick with an action step for at least a week or two before giving it up if it is not working for you.

One change in your lifestyle might not provide any noticeable result. It doesn't mean that you should abandon that change. Unless it is something that doesn't make any difference *and* is also very hard for you to keep up, it is essential to stack up changes and new habits as you keep working on your sleep, so that after a while, the combination of all those changes will bring noticeable results.

Keep in mind that our habits, even the most harmful, are always serving a purpose in our daily life. Though this purpose is not necessarily the one we want or one that is beneficial, habits are serving us in one way or another. Otherwise, we would not have those habits in the first place and it would not be as challenging to change them. For example, checking social media in the middle of the night is an objectively bad habit when it comes to sleep, but maybe it helps us feel more connected and reinforces our sense of safety and community. Remembering this will help you be less frustrated with yourself when you find it hard, or impossible, to change certain habits that you know perfectly well are harmful. Give yourself grace if you want to succeed.

An excellent way to look at this habit-changing process is to consider that everything you are doing is an experiment. The goal is to learn something from each change you make that will help you reassess and move forward. If you decided to go for a 30-minute walk five nights per week, but you can't figure out a way to fit them into your schedule, don't see this as a failure. Look at it as a sign that you are too busy to take that step right now. You might have to reassess this step and try something slightly different. For example, you could start with a 10-minute walk five nights per week or for a 30-minute walk two nights per week. Simultaneously, you could look at your weekly schedule and see where you could carve a bit of room to free up a few minutes at night.

If you have too many action steps to work on, you will lose your focus and eventually quit. Don't set yourself up for failure. Only pick a couple of changes (action steps) at once. Of course, you might

not see results within one week. Still, once you have one healthy habit implemented and relatively secure, you can move to the next one, and little by little, you will build up a new lifestyle where sleep is a priority and you are rested and energized every morning.

Since I don't recommend working on too many steps at once, you might wonder why the Winning Sleep Plan Tracker has so many lines available to record the changes you want to implement. It is because sticking to an action step for a week won't make it become a natural part of your life. When a recently acquired habit seems to work for you, you will need to keep it on your tracker for several more weeks until it becomes something that you "just do," naturally. You will still be able to implement new changes on top of it, but you want to keep newly gained habits top of mind if you don't want them to fall off your radar. Writing them down again in your Winning Sleep Plan Tracker is the best way to maintain them.

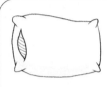

SPECIAL TIP

If you are not sure what goal or action step you should start with, here is a rule you can follow that will allow you to move forward without getting overwhelmed. Pick one harmful habit that you will completely change, and one positive habit that you will reinforce or emphasize.

For instance, if every time you wake up in the middle of the night, you turn on the light and check your work emails, that is obviously impacting your sleep negatively. This is a harmful habit you will ultimately want to eliminate.

If you go on a walk on weekends after dinner and notice that you feel nicely relaxed afterward, you can improve this positive habit by also walking after dinner two additional days of the week. Once you've achieved this, you can further improve by walking every evening.

STEP SIX: TWEAK, REPEAT, AND CELEBRATE!

Once you have filled out one sheet of the Winning Sleep Plan Tracker, reassess and decide on the next steps. Rinse and repeat until you are satisfied with your sleep. You can print as many copies of the Winning Sleep Plan Tracker as you wish. Just like all the other worksheets, you can access this tracker at allonZcoaching.com/sleepitoff with the password SLEEP_IT_OFF. Don't be discouraged by the idea that it might take you a while to get where you want to be. Keep in mind that along the way, your sleep will improve, as will your health and well-being. You could see changes in your weight early in the process, too, and might not need to reach your ultimate goals before you start observing improvements in your blood sugar levels. You have to put in the work for the long term, yes. But most likely, you won't have to wait until the end to experience life-changing results.

Make sure to acknowledge and celebrate your successes. Any improvement, as small as it might be, is still a step in the right direction, and you can be proud of all the effort that you are putting into the process.

CHAPTER SEVEN
25 Real-Life Situations

I don't know about you, but when I'm learning something new, I need examples.

In this book, I have listed a lot of reasons for lack of sleep and given you lots of tips to improve your sleep. For convenience, I have also compiled 100 of them in a checklist with 100 Common Sleep-Killers, which you can download at allonZcoaching.com/sleepitoff. Most likely, it will provide you with plenty of inspiration to help you change your lifestyle successfully.

If you find it intimidating to build your winning sleep plan from scratch, though, don't worry, I have you covered. Over the past years, I have experimented with many sleep improvement strategies, whether for myself or with my clients. To make it easier for you to find action steps that could fit your personal life, I have grouped tips and strategies under various real-life situations that you can relate to.

Here is a list of the 25 real-life situations we will review:

Although you are welcome to do so, you don't need to read all the situations. Just pay attention to the ones most relatable to your own circumstances.

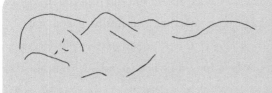

STORYTIME

Barbara didn't understand why she was so tired, even though she slept eight hours every night. A mom of two, she was starting to feel depressed and couldn't help but feel sluggish compared to the other moms at school. She didn't have the energy to be a chaperone on her son's field trips. She didn't feel like hiking with her husband anymore. When her girlfriends decided to go on a girl's getaway in Vegas, she found an excuse because she wasn't sure she could stay up late at night.

In Barbara's mind, she was sleeping enough. She would go to bed at 10 pm and set her alarm for 6 am so that she could have 8 hours of sleep every night. Once she'd walked me through her routine, though, we found out that twice a week, she woke up 45 minutes early to work out. Sometimes her dog would be the one to wake her up at 4 am because he needed to go out and it would take her a little while to fall back to sleep. On Thursday nights, she had a book-club meeting, so she would go to bed around 11 pm, and the wine she drank with the other ladies would usually cause her to be agitated all night and wake up regularly.

Barbara had never really paid attention to these "exceptions" that stole away hours of her sleep. Barbara actually rarely slept for eight hours as she thought she did. She rather averaged six-and-a-half hours. Tracking her sleep and talking through her routine allowed her to identify a few changes to make in her daily habits. She decided to go to bed an hour earlier most nights and to drink less wine during her book club meetings. She also decided to work out on her way home from work instead of early morning. Barbara got her mojo back within a few months, and she is planning on joining her girlfriends' next getaway!

1. If I slept for eight hours every night, I wouldn't have a life anymore.

For most of my clients, this is the main issue. And it was, for many years, my main barrier to sleeping more. There was so much I had to do and so little time to do it. If that sounds like you, start right here before working on any other issue. If you already know how many hours of sleep you need to feel rested, this is great; you can work with that number. If you haven't been able to figure out how much time you need to recharge, you can aim for about eight hours of sleep.

Make sure you allow for the necessary time to sleep as much as you need to. For example, if it usually takes you half an hour to fall asleep, section off 8.5 hours every night rather than just eight. Going to bed earlier than usual is hard because it gives you the feeling that you have no more time for yourself, that you only work, do your chores, and sleep. I get it. I have been there. You can proceed by 10- or 15-minute increments so that you don't have to change your schedule drastically. If you start by adding 15 minutes of sleep every night for one month, you end up with a full extra night's sleep at the end of the month. Once sleeping 15 minutes longer becomes your new standard, you can start adding 15 more minutes the next month.

Taking tiny steps toward my goal is how I went from five hours to almost eight hours of sleep in about three years. If I had tried to add three hours of sleep every night right away, it would have been a nightmare. But doing it little by little did not disturb my schedule as much. It took me a while, but I am well on my way to my ultimate goal of eight-and-a-half hours per night, which I hope to reach by the time I turn 50.

If adding 10 or 15 minutes per night doesn't work for you, you can try going to bed one hour earlier twice a week. Once two nights are doable regularly, you can add another early night. Just work step by step and take your time. This is just like weight loss: if you go too fast, your results won't be sustainable, and you will fall back to your old habits as soon as something gets in the way. Keep in mind that it is about improving, it is not about being perfect.

2. I wake up several times at night for absolutely no reason.

It is essential to know that when we sleep, our brain is still functioning. Not only is our brain doing some clean-up, sorting, and repair. It is also necessary for our brain to stay alert in case we find ourselves in a dangerous situation. Though most of us don't have to watch for predators anymore, there are still reasons to stay alert. There could be a house fire, a break-in, an earthquake, or maybe you are just monitoring the other people in your house, whose safety and well-being you care about.

The fact that our brain is not completely off while we sleep leads to short periods of awakeness throughout the night, which we are not aware of. These micro-awakenings are normal and don't interfere with the quality of our sleep, unless an external or internal trigger, such as noise, light, heat, or having to use the bathroom, wakes us up completely. Since there are lots of micro-awakenings during our night, we have plenty of opportunities to be awakened.

Make sure your sleeping environment can't wake you up when you are experiencing a micro-awakening. That means no blinking lights in the room, no disturbing noise, and a comfortable temperature, appropriate bedding, etc.

You have most likely heard of dust mites and acarids in mattresses, blankets, carpets, etc. They don't bite or sting, but they can lead to a mild allergic reaction that makes you sneeze regularly. If you are in the middle of a micro-awakening and you suddenly feel the need to sneeze, you will wake up, and that could be the end of your night. Another example would be if your bedroom is too hot or too cold. These disturbances might not keep you from falling asleep, but when you go through a normal micro-awakening phase, any discomfort might wake you up for good.

Though reasons to wake up while experiencing a micro-awakening moment are plentiful, they are not all necessarily linked to your environment. They can come from stress – whether positive or negative – from hunger, from our body itching, from the need to use the restroom, etc. This is why it might take a lot of experimenting and good observation skills if you want to identify why you are waking up at night. Keep in mind that micro-awakenings happen regularly during the entire night. If only a couple of these awakenings wake you up completely, it can seriously disturb your sleep cycle, and you can wake up the next morning exhausted. Sometimes, people even have the feeling that they don't sleep at all, even if they actually do.

3. I am tired, but I don't really feel like sleeping.

It is essential to keep your bedroom and your bed reserved for sleeping only. There are only two exceptions to that rule: having sex – it is a great sleep promoter, by the way – and reading a paper book – unless it is full of cliffhangers. If that's the case, try to put your book down in the middle of a chapter to avoid cliffhangers that could keep you reading for hours.

A multi-purpose bedroom is one reason why many teens struggle with sleep. Having your entire world in your bedroom is going to affect your sleep negatively. Most teens and many adults have everything to work, play, or communicate with in their bedroom. Not only can it keep you from wanting to fall asleep, but it also signals to your brain that the bedroom and the bed are not necessarily meant for sleep.

If you have younger children who are also struggling with falling asleep or don't want to go to bed in the first place, storing their toys in a separate room might be helpful. Making the bedroom a place to sleep, with only a few books, some comfort items, and soft light will help them internalize the fact that the bedroom is only for resting and will help them sleep better.

Not everybody can afford to have two separate rooms for each member of a family, but turning one corner of each bedroom into a sleeping nook, with curtains or panels can be sufficient. The idea is to have a separate place and time entirely dedicated to sleep, with no desk, no screens, no toys, and nothing to do but sleep.

Sometimes, we don't realize all the opportunities for activity that our bedroom contains. Do you have a TV in your bedroom? Is your computer right by the bed? Do you do your dumbbell workout in the bedroom or a craft that you enjoy? If you often toss and turn in your bed, try to keep an open mind and move some things away for a couple of months and watch the result.

We are so used to being in crowded environments that it might be hard to notice that our bedroom is keeping our brain alert and busy. Damien Léger, head of the Clinical Sleep and Vigilance Center in Paris, explains that an excellent way to see whether our bedroom needs purging is to take a picture. It makes it easier to spot unnecessary objects and the things that keep us connected to our daily activities rather than putting us in a sleeping mindset. If looking at the picture is not sufficient for you, look at it with someone who has never been in your bedroom and will bring a critical and enriching perspective.[1]

4. I share the bed with my Great Dane; I am exhausted.

There are many good reasons why pet parents would want to share the bed with their beloved pets, and if that's your case, you are definitely not alone. Unfortunately, even if it makes your dog or your cat the happiest pet on earth, chances are it is not helping you rest. Maybe your big dog is taking all the room? Although even the smallest animal can take up a great deal of the bed when it turns sideways! Maybe your puppy can't hold its pee longer than five hours. Is your cat walking all over you in search of warmth and a cuddle? Or is it meowing for food at the crack of dawn?

When I first started sleeping on the couch in my living room, I would wake up every morning around 4 am, and almost every single time, our cat would be right there, looking at me with a blasé look before walking directly to the window sill where he would spend the rest of the night. I assumed that his walking around was waking me up and didn't know what to do about it. But then, once I paid better attention to his routine, I realized that it was actually his eating dried food in the adjacent kitchen that woke me up every morning. He would come in from outside, chew his food, and then walk through the living room. I moved his dry food down to the basement. He kept his routine, but his walking through the living room was not enough to wake me up when his chewing had not put my brain on high alert. Some mornings, I would find him next to me on the couch, and that had not disturbed me at all, either.

If your pet is ruining your sleep, it is important to define precisely the reasons why it keeps you awake. Then, list with a very open mind all the measures you could take to make things different. You can use the Obstacles & Solutions worksheet to do that, with a specific focus on your pet. Once you have a list of solutions, find out solutions that you can implement easily. My guess is that there won't be many, otherwise, you would have solved the problem long ago. But if you find a couple, go ahead and take action. For the other solutions, the ones that seem impossible or cruel (like forbidding access to your room, which would lead to your dog whining all night), it is important to direct your attention to your pet, rather than on your sleep. Could your buddy need more exercise during the day? Or would they feel less lonely in the basement if they had a companion? Could they be trained to sleep on their own bed in your bedroom, rather than together with you?

Talking with your veterinarian is also a good idea. They hear about such situations all the time, and they also hear from people who have found solutions. They know a lot and could help you figure out ways to make things better while keeping your pet happy and safe.

5. I keep tossing and turning; it gets on my nerves.

Don't stay in bed if you can't sleep. You don't want your bedroom to be full of brain solicitations, but you also don't want your bed to become a place where stress is high and frustration creeps in. You want your bed to be the place where you relax and sleep.

If you spend too much time in your bed when you have trouble sleeping, you will become anxious and agitated, and you will start over-thinking. This won't help you sleep, and you will get even more frustrated, which will perpetuate the problem.

Reducing the time spent lying awake in bed is one tool used in Cognitive Behavioral Therapy (CBT) when patients are trying to reduce insomnia or get off sleep medication. The goal, in this case, is to get a more specific idea of how much time you are actually sleeping and spend only that time in your bed for a few days. For instance, if someone is used to spending eight hours in bed but sleeps for only five hours, they would start staying in bed for only five hours. Of course, because of insomnia, they won't sleep five hours, but chances are they will sleep relatively more than before – not if we count the hours they sleep, but if we calculate how much time they sleep compared to the time spent in bed. For instance, if they lie in bed for five hours, they might get around four hours of sleep. Four hours of sleep out of five hours in bed is 80%. This is a better ratio than sleeping five hours when spending eight hours in bed, which would be only about 60% of the time spent in bed and would lead to more frustration. After a few days, people who use that method end up being so exhausted that they start sleeping a little more, until they end up sleeping the whole time they spend in bed. That's when they can start spending a bit more time in bed. Proceeding this way, slowly, helps increase the time they sleep while reducing the time they lie around getting frustrated and anxious. We talked earlier about how the fear of not sleeping can feed insomnia. CBT directly addresses that problem. We will talk more about Cognitive Behavioral Therapy in situation #10.

You might be confused, though, because I have been telling you all along to allocate enough time to your sleep and aim for about eight hours. Now I am telling you the exact opposite! Here's the thing: if you think you need eight hours of sleep but only sleep five hours every night, one part of your action plan will be to remove all the obstacles to your sleep and make sure you meet the "five sleep requirements" listed in chapter four. The other part of your action plan will be to make sure you don't start stressing too much about sleep and especially about sleep deprivation.

Making sure you don't stay in bed for hours while not sleeping is important. You can, for instance, decide that if you can't fall asleep after about 30 minutes, you will get up and do something else. Nothing too exciting, of course. No screen, no bright lights, nothing that gets you thinking, excited, or alert. Ideally, you will do something pretty boring, such as reading a non-captivating book. You can also do something that will promote sleep, like relaxation, stretching, or gentle yoga. Make sure you have all those activities planned ahead of time so that when you decide to get up instead of staying in your bed at night, you don't have to think hard about what you could do. Just get up and do what you had planned on doing. If you go to bed with a list of back-up plans, you will stay on autopilot more or less and will be able to get "active" without activating your brain too much.

Be careful not to shift your daily chores to night time, though. You don't want to find yourself in a situation where if you don't get up, you will fall behind on your chores. Choose activities that you might not do otherwise, slightly useless, if possible. And of course, make sure those activities are not too enjoyable so that you won't look forward to them.

6. I don't know what to eat to sleep better.

It would be way too long to go into the details of what food does to our body, how it affects our hormones, our brain function, and everything else. The food we put in our body has a tremendous influence on how we feel, how we function during the day, and of course, how we sleep. This book is not a nutrition guide, so I will keep it short, but based on science and my experience with clients, I can provide you with a few tips and strategies to make sure your food is not what keeps you from sleeping well, as is the case for so many people I have the privilege to work with.

By now, you have most likely filled out your Daily Journal (chapter six). Chances are that you have noticed patterns, foods that keep you from sleeping well, or foods that make you wake up in the middle of the night because you are sweaty, agitated, or need to use the bathroom.

A few signs that might show that your food intake is not helping your sleep could be that you have puffy eyes in the morning, acid reflux, cramps, headaches, night sweats, bad breath, bloating, white tongue, or feel very gassy.

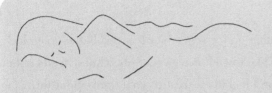

STORYTIME

For Cheryl, the favorite meal of the day was dinner. She would stop by the grocery store on her way home from work and buy fresh produce and other ingredients to prepare a delicious meal for herself and her partner every night. It was healthy, homemade, mostly with whole foods. Nothing extravagant. Often grilled meat or baked fish, some vegetables, and a starch such as pasta, rice, or bulgur. She would also have a side salad, a chocolate truffle for dessert, and a glass of wine while preparing dinner, which she would finish during the meal.

Cheryl had no issue falling asleep, but her nights were interrupted with severe hot flashes. She would wake up drenched in sweat and often had to change her nightgown in the middle of the night and go sleep in the guest room because her sheets were soaked. Cheryl assumed that there was nothing she could do about it and that perimenopause was the culprit. By the same token, she took it for granted that hormonal changes were the reason for the extra pounds she had piled up over the past two years. Cheryl wanted to work with me to lose a bit of weight in her mid-section. She didn't mention her sleep at all until I asked her about it. She was resolved to live with it until her hormones finally settled down.

Cheryl is a driven business owner. I challenged her to eat only a bowl of soup or a light salad for dinner for two weeks, with a piece of fruit for dessert. Of course, she had to make adjustments to her breakfast and lunch, otherwise, she would have been starving. She rose to the challenge and the results were impressive. Within two weeks, the night sweats had almost completely vanished. She would still sometimes wake up soaked in the morning, but it was not enough to wake her up at night. Her hormones had little to do with poor sleep. Too much food and a labored digestion were actually her main issues.

Keep in mind that fatty foods are harder to digest than fruits, vegetables, and lean protein. Also, spicy foods can raise your body temperature, so you might want to limit their intake for dinner.

We are all very different, and we don't have the same nutritional needs, but there are a few rules that often work well for many people, and you might belong to that group of people. So, when it comes to food and beverages, here are a few tweaks that you can try to implement to see whether it helps you sleep better.

- **Keep your dinner light**

Avoid fatty meals, meat, and deli for dinner and rather go for vegetables (especially the green leafy ones) and lean protein (mostly plant-based). If you like to end on a sweet note, choose fruits rather than decadent desserts and sweet treats. If fruits don't feel like a treat to you, think about throwing a bunch of frozen berries in the blender with a little almond or coconut milk. You will get delicious ice cream. Frozen chunks of banana work really well, too. Easy, healthy, and delicious.

- **Have dinner about two to three hours before bedtime**

Trying to sleep on a full stomach might be challenging. You don't want to be starving when you go to bed, because that might keep you from relaxing and falling asleep, but making sure you don't eat too close to bedtime will make a sizeable difference. Finishing your meals at least two to three hours before bedtime is a good bet. If you are used to eating later, you could also eat an apple just before hitting the mattress. It might help you adjust more easily to an earlier dinner.

- **Let your meal get you in a sleepy mood**

This is not really food-related, but you could also try to have candlelight dinners even when there is no special occasion. This will let your brain understand that it is time to shut down. It is also essential to avoid hot topics or serious discussions at dinner time so that you don't raise your stress level.

- **Eat slowly and focus**

Sit down, grab some silverware, and spend at least 30 minutes enjoying your meal. If you take your time, you will chew your food well rather than gobbling up mindlessly, and this will help tremendously, not only with digestion but also with the amount of food you will end up eating. Since being overweight also affects sleep quality, eating slowly might help to keep portions in check and thus lead to weight loss if that's what you need. Of course, it is not quite that simple, but eating slowly is part of an approach that has proven to help with weight loss. Think about putting your fork down between two bites. You can also bring one course at a time to the table rather than putting everything on your plate at once. For instance, start with a bowl of lettuce, a sliced tomato, or a light vegetable soup; once you are done and everybody else around you is done, serve the protein, vegetable, and maybe a small quantity of starch. When your plate and everybody else's plate is clean, if you are still hungry, go for seconds of vegetables until you feel satiated. If you are eating with others, never move to the next course until everyone is done. Eating with someone rather than eating alone can also help slow down the pace because you will talk and hopefully won't do so with your mouth full. So think about rallying your family or a few friends and colleagues, whether you meet in person or virtually, now that we have all become experts in video conferencing.

• **Don't drink alcohol at night (not even a small glass of wine)**

You might think that alcohol doesn't affect your sleep since you only drink a glass of wine when

DID YOU KNOW?

The French eat their meals in three or four courses, all the time. Lunch or dinner, celebratory or weeknight meal, it doesn't make any difference. It doesn't mean that we eat only gourmet meals, though. It is just that we don't serve our food all at once. We stage things, and, as a result, our meals last longer. What happens when you do that is that by the time you have finished eating, your brain has registered that you are full, and you feel satiated. One consequence of eating too fast is feeling deprived because your brain didn't get the message that your stomach was full. When your meals last longer, you feel satisfied and end up eating less. You, too, can eat "the French way."

Sean, one of my clients, tried that strategy after plateauing for months in his weight loss. He had even gained some weight back at the beginning of the 2020 COVID-19 quarantine. A few weeks after we started working together, he decided to eat his meals "the French way" and was astonished that making his meals last 30 minutes instead of 10 minutes made the scale tip again in the right direction.

you come home from work or when you are getting dinner ready. Plus, wine might help you relax and unwind. Unfortunately, you might be wrong. I am not telling you never to drink alcohol again, but if sleeping is an issue for you and you are committed to change that fact, experimenting with a dry month is a good idea. I am pretty sure that you will see some difference in your sleep patterns if you go for several weeks with no alcohol at all, and if that's not the case, at least you will know. Once again, be very honest with yourself and listen to your body.

- **Do not eat or drink anything that has a stimulating effect**

Coffee, tea, energy drinks, caffeinated soda... It is evident that anything containing caffeine should be discontinued at night. What might not be as obvious is that I am not talking only about night time here. As we have seen in chapter five, caffeine can remain in your body for more than 12 hours, so if you are struggling with sleep, don't forget to question that morning cup of coffee that you have every day. Again, I am not saying "no more coffee" ever. But maybe you should try to go three or four weeks without coffee and see if it affects your sleep.

Now, what about the small square of chocolate that you enjoy every night? Chocolate is a stimulant, so is it worth it? Again, there is no one-size-fits-all answer here. You have to decide for yourself, and often, you need to experiment first before you have all the data to help you make a decision. For me, it only takes one square of dark chocolate after dinner to keep me from falling asleep. Now that I know it, I make informed choices. It doesn't mean that I never eat chocolate at all, but I usually keep it for nights when I know I can sleep in the next day, or I eat it during the day.

If you are a smoker, you might not know that nicotine is a stimulant and leads to the release of adrenaline, dopamine, and glucose into the body.[2] Nicotine can also have a depressant effect, but that is not as systematic. So, if you are used to smoking a cigarette right before bed and have trouble falling asleep, I suggest that you refrain from smoking after dinner for a week or two and see what happens.[3]

- **Don't skip meals during the day**

Do you remember when we talked about how your brain needs to feel safe for you to go into deep sleep? That was in chapter four. Your body also needs to feel safe, and one way to make your body feel *unsafe* is to *not* eat your meals at relatively regular intervals. Skipping meals will rarely benefit your health, weight loss, performance, or sleep. Eating at regular times is part of having that comforting routine we already talked about. It allows your body to adjust to a schedule and rely on it. When your body cannot rely on regular food intake, it will be stressed out, and it will release more cortisol. As we have seen, cortisol is one of the hormones that make us alert and awake. We don't want too much of it released regularly or it will impact our sleep negatively.

- **Sip water all day**

Just as your body needs to be nourished, it needs to be hydrated. Water is THE ideal way to stay hydrated. It is important to sip water all day rather than drink large amounts just before bedtime.

You don't want water to interfere with your ability to stay in bed all night because you have to run to the bathroom. Drinking small amounts of water all day long will allow you to keep that water and benefit more from it than if you were drinking a large glass at once and then nothing for several hours. That's what we call gastric emptying. When our stomach is full of liquid, it wants to empty itself. So sipping water regularly keeps us hydrated better because the liquid is not evacuated right away.

• **Drink a warm glass of milk or non-caffeinated tea before bed**

Make sure you won't have to get up three times during the night to go to the bathroom, but drinking a cup of warm milk or herbal tea before bed might help you sleep better. Certain types of tea have calming effects (chamomile, for instance), and milk also contains tryptophan, the amino acid we mentioned in chapter six, which is a prerequisite to serotonin production and thus, melatonin release. Even though the quantity of tryptophan in a glass of milk might not be relevant to helping us sleep, the ritual of taking a break while enjoying a delicious cup of warm milk before bed might help you relax and get your body and brain in the mood for a good night's sleep.

When it comes to food intake and beverages, there is much more, of course. I cannot review everything in this book, but if you feel that you have tried all the above strategies and don't know what to do next to tweak your food intake, it might be worth working with a professional who could help create a plan with you to address your needs and circumstances. I have seen several clients who had given up carbohydrates while following a high-protein/low-carb diet that would supposedly help them lose weight. Unfortunately, several of them ended up struggling with sleep and didn't know why. Complex carbohydrates, found in whole grains, beans, legumes, or vegetables, can help increase our serotonin levels and lower our cortisol levels. As a result, a diet lacking complex carbohydrates might represent an issue for those who struggle with sleep. Including non-processed plant-based food in our dinner can do wonders. On the other end, adding processed carbohydrates such as bread, pastries, or prepackaged meals could make it much harder to sleep well.

An extra tip, while you are adjusting your food intake, would be to go for a leisurely walk after dinner. It will not only help with digestion but will also help you relax and unwind from the day (as long as your neighborhood is safe), bring your core body temperature down, and expose you to the declining light outside. Just like the warm cup of milk or tea mentioned above, a gentle stroll after dinner can also become a ritual that tells your body: "We are now getting ready for bed; be prepared."

7. I don't have a very active life; I'm not sure what to do.

We all know that after a night that was not restful, we won't be as productive during the day. Unfortunately, we tend to forget that after a day when we haven't used all our vitality, it will also be harder to enjoy a good night's sleep. Considering that our lives are becoming less active physically and more stressful, it makes sense that our sleep suffers.

Research has shown that sleep and exercise have substantial positive effects on one another and that being physically active can help mitigate the impact that a sedentary and stressful life has on our sleep. Among many other things, exercise has proved to help with stress, depression, and anxiety, but also with weight, diabetes, and many other chronic diseases. One of the many known reasons why physical activity helps us sleep better is that it increases tryptophan and helps with the release of serotonin, which, we have seen many times already, is a precursor to melatonin, the sleep hormone.[4]

Endurance sports performed outdoors seem to be the ones with the most sleep-inducing effects, but with physical activity, just as with food, caffeine, and pretty much anything else involved in our sleep, there is no cookie-cutter approach. It is necessary to find what works best for you. If you don't know what workout would be best, here are a few pointers.

Choose a workout you enjoy. Ideally, what you choose makes you happy while you do it. It seems obvious, but if you look at what most of us do for exercise, this is a criterion that doesn't often come into the equation. Yet it is probably the most important! Being physically active doesn't have to equate to giving all you've got on a treadmill. Gardening is physical activity; playing with your dog is physical activity; walking is physical activity.

Sometimes, the exercise you choose is not highly enjoyable, but there is something about it that you truly appreciate. Maybe it is the way you feel when you are done. Perhaps it is the image it gives of yourself. Or it is the people you are doing it with, whom you otherwise never get to see. Maybe it is your only chance to be outdoors, or alone, or to listen to music. Whatever it is for you, there *must* be something specific you look forward to or gain from your workout; otherwise, you won't be able to maintain your exercise routine.

When you choose a workout, make sure it doesn't require too much of the resources you don't have. If you are super busy and time is your most scarce resource, make sure that your workout is not too time-consuming. Otherwise, you will always find reasons not to fit it into your busy schedule, and even when you make room for exercise, you will always feel resentful about not doing something else. If it is money that you are lacking and you pick a workout that's not free or super cheap, there will be times when you won't be able to afford exercising. And when you can afford it, you will feel guilty that you are not spending your money elsewhere.

Time and money are often the things we struggle the most with, but maybe your case is different. Whatever it is that you don't have much of, make sure that your new workout routine doesn't make you second guess yourself every time you exercise.

Ideally, you will want to work out without knowing you are working out. Whether you call it "commuting," or "fun with friends," or "walking the dog," if you do the things that you *have* to do in life or that you *want* to do in life, and those things are good workouts, you will end up living an active life naturally. Physical activity will be a given, and you won't have to worry about carving time for the gym or a run. You will become "unconsciously" active, and that will help tremendously with your sleep.

When my husband and I first moved to the United States in 2000, we lived in a South Jersey suburb. I would do what I had always done in Europe: leave the car home when running my errands and walk to the stores. Regularly, a vehicle would pull over and ask me if my car had broken down. Why would I walk otherwise? I admit that it was not the most enjoyable experience, without proper sidewalks and an awkward feeling of insecurity and misfit while strolling through a suburban sprawl. I tried riding my bike, but that didn't feel safe either. So, I did like everyone else around me: I started to use the car even for short distances and became gradually less active and more stressed out. I don't think it is a coincidence that this time of my life is also the time when sleeping was the most difficult. Of course, I had two young children to care for in those years, and that didn't help. But having such a sedentary lifestyle definitely made the matter worse. By the time we moved to the city and settled in a beautiful, walkable, and safe neighborhood of Seattle, I had lost the habit of walking everywhere but was eager to pick it up again.

Just like everything else, things didn't happen overnight. I started walking within a half-mile radius, and only when it was not raining – which is not as rare as you might think! Thanks to the steep hills of Seattle, my daily life became much more active than before, and that quickly lead to a stronger body and better stamina. Nothing exceptional but enough to start riding my bike, with my toddler in the back, when it took too long to walk. The tipping point for me was when my first grader, in an attempt to "stop hurting the planet" as she put it, decided that she would not let me drive her to school anymore. She wanted to walk or ride her bike, no matter the weather or circumstances. Seven years later, as a middle schooler, she has broken that promise only once. The school was only half a mile away; distance was not an issue. But her decision helped me change my mindset and dismiss driving altogether, even when rain was pouring and wind was blowing. This is how I started walking or riding my bike more and more often, longer distances as well, until I would only consider taking the car if I had to get on the highway. For everything else, biking was perfect, whether to go to the store with saddles bags or to go to professional meetings with a change of clothes in my backpack. People around me know me for that, now. They see me ride, walk, or run rain or shine. I don't go to the gym and don't work out much per se, but I am active every day, and that is enough to keep me fit, happy, and balanced. I rarely walk or ride for the sake of it. It is always to go somewhere. Most of the time, it doesn't take much more time than driving, considering the traffic and parking nightmares in Seattle. All it takes is some planning and mindfulness. That comes easy to me, as opposed to having to carve time out of my day for a typical workout.

Of course, walking and riding everywhere is not a solution for everyone. It requires some logistics and a high tolerance for bad hairdos. Plus, most importantly, you need to enjoy riding and feel safe doing so. Find what works for you, keeping in mind that if you struggle with sleep and have a sedentary lifestyle, it might be foolish to expect an improvement unless you drastically increase your level of daily physical activity.

For middle-aged and elderly adults, exercise improves sleep quality and sleep duration regardless of the mode and intensity of the activity, and even more so in populations suffering from a disease.[5] So when you are trying to increase your level of physical activity, don't worry too much about what you do and when you do it. Just keep in mind that one thing that will hinder melatonin production is keeping our body temperature too high by working out too hard just before bedtime. If you want to get a good sweat, it might be best to do that earlier in the day and keep your evening low key, with a stroll outside or a gentle yoga routine before bedtime.

8. I would sleep just fine if it weren't for my partner.

Sleeping in separate beds or separate rooms carries a stigma, and this is a decision you will have to make for yourself. It is commonly believed that sleeping in the same bed is best for the "health" of a couple. It might be. Unless one party involved ends up sleep-deprived and resentful. Sometimes, it is even both partners who suffer.

Have you ever witnessed the animosity at breakfast time when one spouse hasn't been able to sleep because the other was snoring? And more often than not, the snorer's sleep suffered as well from being shaken out of sleep or being hit in the ribs throughout the night. I grew up witnessing those morning fights between my parents, and then between friends and relatives experiencing the same issues. Early on, it was clear to me that sleeping together had absolutely nothing to do with the health of a couple. Intimacy is one thing. Sleeping is another.

You know it by now: I am a light sleeper. For many years, when sleep was not a priority in my life, having my husband snoring lightly next to me was not an issue. I would pick a book and read until I was sufficiently exhausted to fall asleep, finally. But once I committed to sleeping more, even having him breathe next to me became a problem. I had to sleep alone. I resisted the idea, though. Just like taking a baby into your bed doesn't have the favor of most parenting gurus, sleeping in separate rooms raises a lot of questions, and when I mentioned the idea to a few friends, their reaction was one of worry. Were we having relationship issues? Were we a couple in trouble? Their questions and remarks bled on me: was it normal that I wanted to sleep away from him? Were we having marriage issues that I didn't want to acknowledge? For several months, I tried to run with the hare and hunt with the hounds. I would go to bed with my husband every night, and after two hours of desperately trying to sleep, would move to the couch for the rest of the night. I have heard a lot of stories where the snorer is the one sent to the couch. I didn't want to resort to that solution since it would have led to both of us having our sleep disrupted instead of only me, and it doesn't solve the problem for the long term. Gradually, I started moving to the couch sooner, until I realized that it was useless to even get in bed with my husband in the first place when sleeping was my only goal. Indeed, once I became frustrated and resentful because I couldn't sleep, it became very hard to relax, whether I stayed next to him or moved to the living room. That's when I made the couch my new bed. It was not necessarily ideal and required that the family adjust to this unique setting – my husband, of course, but also my children. No one could use the living room once mom was ready for sleep, and I had to give up the thought of having a bedroom for myself – we don't have a guest room. But believe me, it was worth the initial work, and with open communication, the change ended up being sustainable in the long term and beneficial to all of us. Years later, I am still getting eight hours of good sleep on my couch most nights, unless one of the family members is out and I can take their bedroom, which feels like a real treat. When I ask my husband how this decision has changed our lives, his answer is straightforward: "We both sleep better!"

When you tell people that you are sleeping away from your partner, many assume conjugal struggles. It is fine. You don't have to justify yourself to the world, or even reassure them. The only people involved here are you and your partner. It is essential to discuss the issue openly and experiment with a solution without hurting anyone's feelings in the process. Sleeping away from your partner takes work if you want to protect intimacy and love. It is hard to give up time together that you may not otherwise have. For a couple struggling with intimacy, sleeping together may be all they have to connect, and it will take some creativity to stay close when sleeping in different beds. A split mattress might be a good alternative if your sleeping partner is restless rather than loud. It is very common for couples in Europe to sleep on two separate mattresses that make up a king bed. Two twin beds in the same room are also an option to consider if your partner keeps waking you up throughout the night because of their restlessness or sleep schedule.

Define your priorities and what is best for you and your family: sleeping well away from each other, or being sleep-deprived together. This is a decision that only you can make and then slowly work toward what might be a suitable compromise. As always, take your time, experiment, and make sure to share your motivation and your profound why with the person who will have to sleep alone if you go this route.

One thing to always keep in mind is that sleep has nothing to do with intimacy. You can have a happy and satisfying sexual life without spending all your nights with your partner. If you wake up three times per night to cuddle, improving your sleep is probably not your priority right now. But for anyone else, let me tell you that sleeping in separate beds can really reinforce intimacy and even feelings between lovers. It is something worth trying for a little while, without guilt and without shame. You will quickly see whether it is for you or not, and then you can decide. Remember that only you and your partner are experts in your relationship – not your mom, your counselor, or your best friend.

9. There is so much noise around; it is impossible to sleep well.

Noise can be a real issue for many people. There are certain disturbances that we can get rid of relatively easily, and others that we have no control over.

Using earplugs can often be the solution. Depending on how much noise reduction you want, you can use wax earplugs (almost complete noise cancellation) or soft earplugs (dull but don't eliminate noise). If you haven't tried earplugs yet, I encourage you to try them as they help muffle the sounds that wake you up. Not all earplugs are alike, though. Depending on their color and shapes, they won't filter the same level of noise and will also fit differently in your ear. It is worth experimenting with a few different options until you find earplugs that fit well. The only ones that work for me are specially designed for smaller ear canals; I can't find them in my local pharmacy and have to order them online.

If earplugs don't work for you, a trick that could help is to add white noise to your sleeping environment. White noise can come from a fan, a fountain, or an app on your phone. I have been using the free application "White Noise Lite" with success, and several of my clients have also experienced the benefits of listening to torrential rain pouring or crickets chirping all night. White noise includes a wide range of sound waves. It is continuous and covers other sharp noises that would usually alert your brain and arouse it. Avoid using white noise regularly to keep from becoming dependent on it. Using a white noise app on your phone might keep you awake by introducing another piece of technology that emits blue light and can make falling asleep more difficult, though. So, as usual, make sure you know why you are using one strategy over another and always monitor the results carefully.

10. My mind is racing, and I can't shut it down.

Have you ever gone to bed and all you can think of are the tasks that you need to accomplish the next day? Things like grocery lists, meetings, clients you need to get back to, relatives you need to call, etc. The problem is, reviewing these activities repeatedly will keep your brain from slowing down before bed. One simple way to let your brain rest is to take a piece of paper (not your phone) and write down everything you have to do, say, or think about the next day. Once the to-do-list is on paper, you won't have to keep its contents in your brain, and you can let go of these stressors. Research has shown that the more detailed the list, the better because it reassures you that you won't forget anything.

You can take this even further by writing every single thing that is on your mind. Write not only a to-do list, but add all your worries, thoughts, goals, and anything else you are thinking of. We call this a brain-dump. Writing everything down will reassure you, and it will be easier to fall asleep. When you wake up, you can read what you wrote and start where you left off.

If a brain-dump is not your style, below are a few other techniques (presented in alphabetical order) that some of my clients find helpful to empty their minds and unplug.

- **Breathing**

Breathing is a powerful tool to combat stress and help you relax at night when your brain is hyperactive. Exhaling for longer than we inhale helps our parasympathetic system kick in, which, as we have seen in chapter four, is one of the five keys to good sleep. Research has even revealed that a mindful slow-breathing session performed at bedtime may "enhance restorative processes at the cardiovascular level during sleep."[6]

Many of my clients, once they have used breathing to relax at night, end up taking several short "breathing breaks" during the day because it allows them to be focused and clear-headed.

Relaxation breathing helps calm down your autonomic system. This system controls automatic body functions such as heartbeat, blood pressure, swallowing. People who practice deep breathing regularly become very good at calming down in just a few minutes.

There are many techniques available to you when you want to practice relaxation breathing. Look online for belly breathing, box breathing, diaphragmatic breathing, or three-part breathing and find a technique that resonates with you. Try several of them out and see what happens. You can even come up with your own combination of methods.

Christopher Hill, Doctor of Chiropractic, shares with us his favorite breathing technique for stress relief and good sleep. It is effortless, and you can do it anywhere, anytime, and especially at night if you are battling insomnia. All you have to do is breathe with the following numbers in mind: 5/5/10/5. Five seconds inhale; hold for five seconds; ten-second exhale; hold for five seconds. Repeat a few times. "This cadenced breathing technique can have a direct impact on your cardiovascular system and will drive the stress hormones down," says Hill.[7]

You can use the technique any time during the day when you feel stress coming up, but if you also make it part of your bedtime routine, you will hopefully see a change in the quality of your sleep.

- **Cannabidiol, aka CBD oils**

CBD stands for cannabidiol, a compound present in cannabis, just like tetrahydrocannabinol, the well-known THC. CBD and THC are both cannabinoids. One fundamental difference between the two compounds is that THC is responsible for the "high" experienced when using cannabis, whereas CDB is not.

According to a report from the World Health Organization, "In humans, CBD exhibits no effects indicative of any abuse or dependence potential.... To date, there is no evidence of health-related problems associated with the use of pure CBD."[8]

According to a few studies cited by the American Sleep Association and the Harvard Health Blog, CBD might be a way to help decrease anxiety and manage insomnia.[9]

Keep in mind that some CBD oils might still contain THC, though, and when that is the case, they may only be sold where the use of marijuana has been legalized. Furthermore, there have been side effects associated with the use of CBD oils, and because they are mostly sold as supplements rather than medicine, regulations are pretty lax (see chapter nine for more information on supplements.) For these reasons, I encourage you to talk to your health care provider and review the potential side effects that you could experience and also how CBD could interfere with the medications you are already taking.[10] I have not used CBD myself and don't suggest that you do, but like other alternative solutions presented in this chapter, it might be something to look into and learn more about.

- **Cardiac Coherence**

Our heart and brain are in constant communication. For example, the brain sends messages to the heart, for instance, to speed up our heartbeat to respond to a stressful situation. We have all experienced our heart racing when we are scared or feel a strong emotion. What we are not as aware of, though, is that our heart also sends messages to our brain and is quite talkative.

Cardiac coherence, also called psychophysiological coherence, is when the various systems in our body such as digestion, respiration, brain activity, immune response, nervous systems, and hormonal systems are all synchronized to the regular rhythm of our heartbeat. According to Lew Childre, founder of the HeartMath Institute, this coherence provides a feeling of inner peace and serenity, allowing us to respond in a calmer and more composed way to external stress. It also makes it easier to fall asleep and enjoy a prime-quality deep sleep.[11]

Cardiac coherence can be promoted by using slow and deep breathing while directing our attention to our heart to slow our heartbeat and consequently slow all of our other systems. This technique has been used by the Navy to help US Armed Forces regulate their emotions and manage stress and trauma. It is a straightforward technique that you can use at any time, and especially at night. For more information about the method, you can visit the HeartMath Institute website or visit other resources on the internet that will walk you through cardiac coherence breathing.

- **Cognitive Behavioral Therapy**

In 2016, The American College of Physicians (ACP) officially recommended, in the Annals of Internal Medicine, that Cognitive Behavioral Therapy (CBT) become the number one treatment put forward by doctors to manage chronic insomnia.[12]

Cognitive Behavioral Therapy consists of evidence-based practices that bring attention to our thoughts, challenge them, and identify actions and behaviors to be changed. Because sleep hygiene is so vital to good mental health, many therapists will discuss the condition of your sleep throughout your treatment, no matter the original reason for the therapy. This will include all the aspects of sleep that we have reviewed in this book: your bedtime routine, how long it takes to fall asleep, whether you wake up during the night, how rested you feel in the morning, whether you nap during the day, or how many hours per night you allocate to sleep.

When you work with a therapist, you will both decide on a target for your work, assess the behaviors to be changed, and determine any cognitive distortions or distressing emotional responses.

Of course, many people are able to change behaviors around their sleep on their own, and this book is designed to help guide you through the process. "Some things to consider when working on behavior change without a therapist," says Mary Torres, Mental Health Counselor, "are motivation, perfectionism, acceptance, and tolerance of distress."[13]

Here are a few things that Torres recommends you work on if you explore CBT on your own:

Behavioral

- No daytime naps
- Turn off electronics earlier
- Refrain from alcohol
- Purposefully stay up for one night to get very tired on night two (extreme, not recommended for all situations or people)
- Progressive muscle relaxation

Cognitive/emotional

- Pull thoughts away from anxiety and emotions (right brain) and move to science/math/data (left brain) by quoting the periodic table of elements, or doing mental math (e.g., 400-7=393. 393-7=386. 386-7=379. And so on...)
- Pull thoughts away from daytime stress by mentally writing a narrative that is enjoyable (e.g., imagining yourself the hero of an inspiring story...)
- Happy-place mindfulness exercise: picture where you would love to be and engage all five senses (e.g., on a beach with sand between your toes, the smell of the salty air and the

taste of a beach barbecue, the sound of waves crashing, and seeing dolphins jumping in the ocean)

While an experienced coach can be a great help when someone has stalled, continually procrastinates, or needs some accountability, a therapist is an ideal partner when there are underlying mental illnesses, which are outside the scope of practice of a coach and often too difficult to approach alone, such as post-traumatic stress disorder (PTSD) or obsessive-compulsive disorder (OCD).

Most CBT therapists will note their treatment orientation on their website, in their profile on your insurance member portal, or the Psychology Today website. There are so many techniques associated with CBT that you can choose from a variety of therapists. Typically, the best work happens when you connect with your therapist personally. According to Torres, it is essential to approach finding a therapist as you would approach a job interview. "You will spend an hour together at a time, usually for several weeks, so if you don't feel comfortable with a therapist, try another."

- **Hypnosis and Self-Hypnosis**

Some people use hypnosis and self-hypnosis as tools to improve their sleep. Self-hypnosis, just like other relaxation techniques, might not bring miraculous results if it is the only strategy you are using. Still, if it is combined with relevant behavioral changes, it can help you be more successful at fighting stress-induced insomnia.

Hypnosis is a simple guided process that can be used as a segue into a deep and peaceful sleep. The word comes from the Greek word "hypnos," which means "sleep." Don't get confused, though. When you experience hypnosis in a therapeutic setting, there is no sleeping involved, just a feeling of deep relaxation. When in a state of hypnosis, theta waves occur in the brain, just like in stages one and two of our sleep cycles (see chapter three). These brain waves are much slower than the beta and alpha waves experienced when we are awake and alert. They are still faster than the delta waves of deep sleep, but they allow for a smooth transition into sleep.

According to Anthony Gitch, Board Certified Clinical Hypnotherapist affiliated with the International Certification Board of Clinical Hypnotherapists (ICBCH), "Getting your brain into the theta state is easy; it just takes a little practice. When you practice self-hypnosis, you are focusing on one thought or a variety of thoughts, and there is no wrong way to do it."[14]

Gitch explains that a sleep-inducing self-hypnosis ritual can be as simple as allowing yourself to become comfortable and relaxed. Once you have become relaxed, it doesn't matter what "boring" activity the mind does, such as listening to the sound of a metronome or imagining yourself walking down an endless winding staircase. The idea is to control cognitive overactivity by producing a relaxation response triggered by a phrase or nonverbal cue.[15]

For an easier introduction to hypnosis, consider a self-hypnosis MP3 download. Gitch offers a free download on his website, but there are also lots of audio resources available on the internet, such as a smartphone application called "The Smart Session App" that streams audio from an extensive library of hypnosis MP3s.

• Meditation

According to the Centers for Disease Control (CDC), meditation has grown three-fold in popularity in the United States over the past few years, and more and more people recognize its effectiveness in reducing stress and feeling more centered and balanced.[16] Meditation is the fastest-growing unconventional health practice among adults, and its effects on sleep have been scientifically verified.[17]

One goal of meditation is to eliminate worries about the past or the future and focus fully on the present. It helps you calm down when your mind is racing. Just like self-hypnosis, meditation puts your brain into a state of mental relaxation while still being awake. With meditation, brain waves slow down, and you enter stages one and two of sleep, which makes it much easier to transition into deep sleep.[18]

There are different techniques in meditation, such as moving meditation, mantra meditation, and breath awareness meditation. If you haven't tried meditation yet, you could search online for free applications and videos or grab a beginner's book at your local library to get a feel for what it is and how you can use it. If you can afford it, you could also find a meditation class to join. You would most likely experience success much faster, as long as you found an instructor who fitted your style.

Meditation is simple, but it doesn't mean it is easy. Just like a workout will require your muscles and lungs to work hard, a meditation session, when you get started, will require your brain to work hard. It can be exhausting, so make sure you are not setting the bar too high when you start. Don't feel discouraged if you can't meditate for more than a few minutes at first. It takes time to build stamina. It also takes consistency.

One of the most destructive myths about meditation is that you supposedly have to completely empty your mind. It makes most people give up on meditation because they can't do it. The brain's job is to think, so it is always going to think. The concept of meditation is not to "empty your head" but rather to "let go of your thoughts." That is where the real magic of meditation is in today's busy and distracted world.

If you can, try meditating at the same time every single day, and always in the same place, so it becomes a ritual. Meditating several times per day will help you progress and get results faster. Still, it is not always workable, so remember that any effort you make to improve your sleep and wellness is better than doing nothing. Acknowledge your efforts and be compassionate, always.

•

We will review more stress relief techniques in situation #12. Whatever you experiment with, be open-minded and just explore. It is essential to approach these with a curious mindset. Worst-case scenario, if they don't help you sleep or relax, you will at least know more about them and most likely discover something about yourself.

11. I am anxious about what's going on in the world.

I meet many people who tell me that they become stressed and depressed because of the political climate of our world. If you have been in the habit of watching the news at night or during the day or checking social media to get the latest scoop on local break-ins, it might be a good idea to rethink these habits to eliminate unnecessary stress from your life.

Imagine not watching the news for a week.

What would happen? How would it change the world, and how would it change your life? Would it make a dent in your stress? Take the time to answer these questions and decide whether cutting back on your consumption of news is something you'd like to try. If you can't stomach the idea of not being connected with the world and not knowing what is going on around you, that's perfectly understandable. In that case, you can try to select news sources that emphasize the positive changes in the world. News channels rarely spend much time on altruism and generosity, but you can find documentaries and international reporting that show you a more peaceful and optimistic picture. Try this for a few weeks and see how it affects your stress.

Another way to be selective when it comes to your exposure to world news is to direct your attention to areas where you *do* have some sort of control. Watching the news can be overwhelming and make you feel helpless and scared. Defining where and how you can have an impact is empowering and can help you be "picky" in the type of information you let enter your life. Concentrating on actions is a great way to stay centered and focused.

Becoming familiar with your community through volunteer work can help you see the world from a fresh angle. You will meet some dedicated members of your community and create deep connections that might help you lower your stress level while making you feel safe in your environment. The avenues to reduce stress are endless, but feeling connected and safe among selfless human beings is a great way to keep your hormones balanced, which is a key to good sleep. If anxiety and loneliness are an issue for you, it is worth tackling the problem with an expert. There is help available, but you need to reach out and ask for it.

12. I have a stressful life; there is nothing I can do about it.

Stress builds up as the day goes on, and you might not always be in control of your stressors or able to eliminate them. Plus, it takes time to readjust your lifestyle and mindset to avoid the stressors that can be avoided. I highly recommend that you work on the root causes of your stress. Even though it requires more effort and time, this is how you will get the most sustainable results. Meanwhile, here are some strategies to help you cope with the side effects of your stressors.

Techniques we discussed earlier in situation #10, such as deep breathing, CBD oils, cognitive behavioral therapy, hypnosis, and meditation, can also be used to calm yourself on a regular basis. Let's review a few additional ways to mitigate the effect of stress in your life. The techniques described below can be used regularly in your daily routine to prevent stress in the first place, or on the go, when tension builds up, whether at night or during the day.

• **Acupuncture and Acupressure**

We often think of acupuncture in terms of treating pain, but it can also help with respiratory and digestive issues, as well as hormonal imbalance, stress, and insomnia.

Acupuncture is rooted in the medical theory and practice of China and is over 2,000 years old. According to Nancy Ishii, Licensed Acupuncturist (LAc AEMP), difficulty falling asleep or staying asleep, feeling restless at night, or having vivid dreams that keep us from feeling rested in the morning can be symptoms of imbalances in specific acupuncture channels or organ systems. Ishii explains that "Acupuncture treats these imbalances to promote the body's innate ability to heal. It can decrease inflammation, increase circulation, help balance hormones, reduce pain, and promote relaxation."[19]

There are many styles of acupuncture based on unique cultures, schools of thought, and traditions. Many practitioners use more than one style in their practice. Contrary to popular belief, acupuncture isn't just about the needles. "The needles are used to promote a healing response from the body," says Ishii. Your acupuncturist may also incorporate cupping (suction), moxibustion (warming), tuina (massage), guasha (scraping), qi gong (exercises), or herbal formulas to support your treatment.

Most people find their acupuncturists through word of mouth. You can also find licensed practitioners online through a local acupuncture college, your state department of health, or the National Certification Commission for Acupuncture and Oriental Medicine.[20]

Acupressure, just like acupuncture, focuses on stimulating acupoints in our body. Studies[21, 22] have confirmed the effectiveness of acupressure on the quality of sleep. If you're having trouble sleeping, even if occasionally, Ishii suggests that you relax and press or gently knead each of the following points for three to five minutes at bedtime each night:

Press the "An Mian" (Peaceful Sleep) points toward the back of the neck. To locate, feel for the bony protrusion behind each earlobe. Apply light pressure with your finger just behind the bone.

Press Heart 7 (HT7) "Shen Men" (Spirit Gate). With your palm facing you, flex your wrist, imagine a line from the tip of your pinkie finger to the wrist crease. In the slight dip just below the palm on the pinkie side of the wrist, press or gently knead this point with your thumb.

Press SP6 "San Yin Jiao" (Three Yin Meeting). This point is on the inside of the ankle. Find the highest point of the ankle bone on the inside of the leg. Measure four finger-widths up toward your knee. Just behind the bone of the upper ankle gently apply deep pressure. Do not press during pregnancy.

- **Essential oils**

Harpreet Gujral, program director of integrative medicine at Sibley Memorial Hospital in Washington D.C., explains in an article for the Johns Hopkins University School of Medicine that "Essential oils don't work for everyone, but there's no harm in trying them as long as you use them in a safe way."[23]

Even though further studies are needed to establish their effectiveness, certain essential oils seem to represent a relatively safe alternative to medication, especially in cases of mild insomnia.[24]

There is growing evidence that inhaling lavender might be an appropriate way to help treat mild insomnia and improve sleep quality.[25]

If you want to experiment with essential oils, do so safely and after talking to your doctor, a naturopath, or an aromatherapist, especially if you have allergies, are pregnant or breastfeeding, or take blood thinners or medication to treat high blood pressure.

Essential oils commonly associated with better sleep are lavender, jasmine, chamomile, and bergamot. Keep in mind that not all plants are inoffensive, and don't assume that because essential oils are natural, they are always safe to use.

Using essential oils regularly as part of a bedtime routine might also increase their effectiveness. We have seen in chapter four that bedtime rituals help provide a sense of safety and calm, so even if essential oils are only providing a placebo effect, the benefits of a self-care routine before sleeping will at least help your body relax and pick up the cue that it is time to settle for the night.

- **Massage and self-massage**

Just like acupuncture, we often use massage to alleviate physical pain. But massage therapy can also be helpful to calm and balance our nervous system. As we have seen in chapter four, when we are under physical or emotional stress, the sympathetic nervous system kicks in and keeps us in a state of high alertness that hinders restful sleep.

Elise Kloter, Licensed Massage Therapist (LMT), explains that a variety of massage techniques can help stimulate the parasympathetic nervous system and bring the body to a calmer state.[26] Her observations are confirmed by research. A review of 25 studies testing the impact of massage therapy on stress confirmed that after a professional massage, levels of the stress hormone cortisol were temporarily lower and heart rate had slowed down.[27] Studies have also shown that massage promotes the release of serotonin and oxytocin, among other hormones. If you remember from chapter three, oxytocin is the precursor to the sleep hormone melatonin and is a neurotransmitter that counteracts cortisol.

Some of Kloter's favorite techniques to help her patients with stress are myofascial release, reiki, and craniosacral therapy. Myofascial release is a hands-on technique. It focuses on relaxing contracted muscles throughout the body by applying gentle pressure on the fascia, tissues that wrap around and support our muscles. Since fascia have abundant nerve endings, releasing them can lower your stress level. Kloter also likes reiki for stress reduction. Reiki is a simple and safe method where the practitioner uses their hands to move energy throughout the body. According to Kloter, "reiki can be extremely effective in reducing stress and returning the body to internal stability (homeostasis)." For her, "craniosacral therapy is also a powerful way to calm the nervous system." Craniosacral therapy is a subtle, hands-on technique that releases restrictions in the membranes of the spinal cord while increasing the flow of cerebrospinal fluid between the brain and the base of the spine. As Kloter puts it, "When nerves can function unhindered, the entire body works more efficiently, and stress goes down."

If you decide to look for a potential massage therapist, it is essential that you check their experience and specialty, but also make sure they are licensed and have received the proper training. Certification by the National Certification Board for Therapeutic Massage and Bodywork[28] (NCBTMB), or affiliation to either the American Massage Therapy Association[29] (AMTA) or the Associated Bodywork Massage Professionals[30] (ABMP) is a good place to start if you cannot get a referral directly from your healthcare provider.

On top of regularly working with a massage therapist, if you can afford it, you could also learn how to work with a partner and help each other relax. If that is not an option, you could use self-massage techniques to combat insomnia. Stimulating reflex points on your body to calm the nervous system is an excellent way to start. Kloter's favorite is the solar plexus point on the soles of the feet. Kloter recommends that you access this point in the center of your foot just below the ball of the foot and simply apply pressure to it to induce relaxation throughout your entire body. You can also use your thumb to trace increasingly larger circles in a clockwise direction. Proceed gently, then switch directions. You can also find this point in the middle of the palm of your hand.

Another technique Kloter learned from a Chinese physician while traveling in China involves rubbing the "third eye" 100 times in a clockwise direction before going to sleep. You can find that point between the eyebrows. You can also massage the indentation behind your earlobes in a circular motion for a few minutes.

- **Relaxation**

Even though relaxing at night is the number one condition to deep and uninterrupted sleep, it is not necessarily a natural state to reach when both your body and spirit are restless. A relaxation response doesn't just occur because we want it. It might take practice and a bit of experimentation before you can mindfully relax when you need it the most.

There are many relaxation techniques available to you if you want to practice intentional relaxation. Among others, you can look into the three methods briefly described below:

Autogenic Training

With autogenic training exercises, you direct your attention to sensations of warmth and heaviness in various parts of your body. Not only does autogenic training help reconnect body and soul, but it also keeps the mind from racing from one thought to another and from one worry to the next, as it focuses its energy on physical feelings.[31]

Progressive relaxation

When practicing progressive relaxation, also known as Jacobson relaxation, you focus your mind on tightening and relaxing various muscle groups of your body, one after the other. Often, progressive relaxation is used alongside deep-breathing techniques and guided imagery exercises.[32]

Guided imagery

Guided imagery can be self-directed, or you can listen to a recording. The goal of guided imagery is to concentrate on a pleasant image in your head or an enjoyable story so that your mind can let go of the negative feelings and thoughts that would otherwise keep you awake.[33]

If you think relaxation is something you want to explore, I encourage you to start with one technique and stick to it for at least a week before you switch to another one. It takes practice before you can experience results. When a method doesn't work for you, don't see this as a failure. Continue exploring and experimenting until you find what clicks.

When I was in 12th grade and struggled with sleep as I had never struggled before, my mom made the loving decision to sign me up – and sign herself up as well, for support – for a six-month relaxation course at the local Community Center. It was horrible! Every Monday night, the class would last 60 minutes. To me, it felt like a full hour of completely wasted time. I would come home frustrated and, of course, incapable of falling asleep, beating myself up for not being more responsive to my mom's effort. I was also mad at her for making me do "nothing" for one hour every Monday night when I should have been studying. I wanted to quit. She didn't let me. And I thank her for that today. I still don't do very well with relaxation exercises, guided imagery, or static meditation. But thanks to these relaxation classes, I learned, 30 years ago, how to breathe properly, and it has served me well so far when dealing with stress or when working out. Since then, I have also found out that I can relax much better when my body is moving, whether it is dancing, walking, or the ultimate meditative exercise for me: swimming.

- **Yoga**

Yoga can be very beneficial for stress and anxiety; it affects our nervous system and stress response. Regular yoga practice may help lower cortisol levels and blood pressure and slow down the heart rate. It also increases the production of gamma-aminobutyric acid (GABA), the neurotransmitter that slows down communication between the neurons, as explained in chapter four.[34]

There are many styles of yoga, so be thoughtful when finding one that works well for you. Hot yoga and vinyasa yoga, for instance, will get your heart rate to rise, so it is best to keep them out of your bedtime routine and instead practice them during the day. Hatha and nidra yoga, which focus on postures and mindful breathing, will be more relaxing and will be better choices to help with your sleep.[35] Studies suggest that during yoga nidra, often described as sleep yoga, alpha brainwave activity increases, which is also what happens as we are falling asleep.[36]

According to Tamara Gillest, Certified Yoga Therapist (C-IAYT), even a short yoga practice can pave your way to a better night's sleep, and you don't have to engage in tricky postures that would require athletic abilities or even flexibility.[37] For Gillest, "The key is a slow movement using a slow synchronized breath." She explains that movements can be elementary like sweeping arms, gentle arcs of the body, supported forward bends, and gentle twisting. Doing slow rocking movements of the legs and shoulders often relaxes the body. Taking slow breaths and increasing the length of the exhale has this effect as well, whether you are lying down or sitting up. Wide sweeping arm movements also signal the nervous system to unwind.

For the beginning practitioner, Gillest recommends starting with body sensing in the comfort of your home. Sit or lie down and begin with breath awareness. Mindfully slow the breath down by taking gentle breaths and increasing the length of the exhale. Guide your awareness through your body, starting with your mouth and head (very sensitive areas of the body), and working down to your toes. From here, you can try making some sweeping arm moves and rock your bent legs side to side slowly. Try moving your body slowly and gently. Consider circling your hips, twisting gently side to side, performing forward folds (if your back allows), and squatting, either standing or taking a squat shape on your back with flexed feet to protect your knees. These are all relaxing moves for your nervous system if you perform them slowly and gently.

For Gillest, it is essential to keep in mind that all forms of yoga include being compassionate with yourself, and you need to "Move to feel good, not to create pain. There is no gain in pain." If something hurts, listen to your body and dial back to alleviate discomfort. Your body is smart enough to send you just the right message, and trusting this is vital to overall physical and mental health.

Adding yoga to your daily routine can not only help you achieve better sleep, but it can also improve your quality of life, as suggested by a study published in the Journal of Ayurveda and Integrative Medicine.[38] If you have not yet tried the most commonly used complementary health approach among US adults, now could be a perfect time to start.

• • •

There are many more practices that you can explore to help lower your stress level and set yourself up for sleep success. You could look into Shiatsu, Tai Chi, earthing, energy work, sound therapy, and many more if you feel that such practices might help you reach a calmer state of mind.[39]

One of my quick and easy tricks, when experiencing an uncomfortable thought or emotion (whether it is stress or something else), is to pause and drink a glass of water while visualizing the water taking away the negative feelings and eliminating toxins from the body. Even if you are skeptical of this visualizing exercise, it doesn't hurt to try. Zero in on the cleansing power of water. It will help you slow down, which is so critical when stress kicks in, and it will also keep you hydrated, which is essential for keeping your body's stress level lower. Drinking water regularly not only helps with stress, but it will also help regulate other bodily functions. If you do it for a while, it will become a habit that will help you stay healthy, physically and emotionally. In fact, a symptom of chronic dehydration is depression. It is a good idea to make sure we are drinking water regularly.[40]

Keep in mind that all the above methods can reduce the symptoms of your stress. If you are dealing with chronic stress, it is essential to address its roots rather than just its effects. Self-reflection will be necessary if you want to identify where your stress is coming from and how you can change your life or yourself to beat stress at the source. Coaching and therapy can help a lot with such efforts.

13. I feel anxious at night; I don't know why.

Our sympathetic system needs to quieten down for us to fall asleep and sleep through the night. Many factors affect our sympathetic system, but one of the most important ones, and most often overlooked, is safety. If our brain doesn't feel safe, it will be very hard for us to relax because our nervous system will make sure our brain stays alert and responsive to every single noise, light, or movement that happens in our environment. There is nothing we can do against this instinct for survival, but we can do our best to create a safe environment for sleep.

Many people have experienced success with a weighted blanket. As explained in an article from February 2019 on the Penn Medicine Website, a weighted blanket applies pressure on your entire body, which gives you a feeling of being hugged and helps activate your parasympathetic nervous system. It can help with your feeling more secure in your bed and being more able to relax and let go.[41]

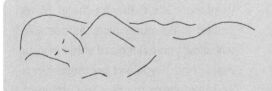

STORYTIME

After a break-up with her boyfriend, Debra found it very hard to relax and sleep through the night. For a long time, she assumed that it was because of the trauma she had experienced from the break-up. As we worked together on reversing her prediabetes, she was also processing the separation with the support of her therapist and gave herself all the compassion she deserved to go through such a painful phase of her life. Unfortunately, even after the painful feelings and emotions were gone, her sleep problem persisted and she still struggled to fall asleep and sleep through the night.

For a while, Debra assumed that loneliness and the heavy silence in her apartment were what kept her awake. But after learning that feeling safe was key for our brain waves to slow down, she realized that she never felt completely secure in her own home because her ex-boyfriend still had the key to the house. He was not a threat to her and would never have harmed her, but the fact that he could come in uninvited kept her in a permanent state of alertness.

Debra changed the locks and, right away, her sleep improved. She felt secure in her bedroom again and knew that no one could come and disturb her sleep at night. Changing the locks was also key (!) to her being able to finally move on and start dating again.

Make sure your bedroom is not an "unsafe" place. If you are worried about someone climbing through the window at any time, you won't relax. Even though you love the fresh air coming in, it might be worth shutting the window or locking the door, for example. Think of any less obvious worries that might linger in the back of your mind: are you slightly worried about your natural-gas furnace being too old? Do you trust your roommate or your pet? Are you 100% sure that the painting over your bed is securely attached? Think about any factors that might make you subconsciously feel unsafe in your bedroom.

Once you find any reason to feel unsafe when you are trying to sleep, make sure you eliminate it or find ways to mitigate it, at least. Otherwise, an excellent deep sleep will never be on your agenda.

Of course, as we have seen before, many areas of our lives create opportunities for feeling unsafe: work, finances, relationships, immigration status, parenting, and many more. It is difficult to eliminate the issues that make us feel insecure. It is essential to identify these factors and start working on them as soon as we can.

> ## SPECIAL TIP
>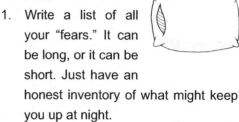
> 1. Write a list of all your "fears." It can be long, or it can be short. Just have an honest inventory of what might keep you up at night.
>
> 2. For each fear, identify the very worst thing that could happen and write it down. Sometimes, doing this is enough to help you relax because you realize that the worst-case scenario is, in fact, not that bad.
>
> 3. Take steps to make sure that the worst-case scenario will not happen. Depending on the situation, you might want to have several back-up plans in place. Often, having these plans written in as much detail as possible will allow you to let go of some of your fears. And if you act on these plans and take steps to solve the problems that are at the root of your worries, you will be in a better place to avoid a lot of emergencies in the future.

No matter what keeps you up at night, looking at your potential problem in a matter-of-fact manner can help ease your stress. Use the Peace of Mind Plan in your workbook to identify sources of insecurity and start creating a prevention plan.

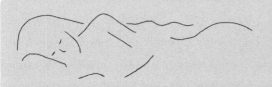

STORYTIME

Elena had a one-hour commute to work every day. Every morning, she would buckle up her twin toddlers in the back, drop them off at her parents' house where her mom would care for them all day, and get on her way to the hair salon where she was styling. She was driving a 16-year-old Santa Fe. She couldn't help but worry that her car would break down and leave her with no way to work, no money to feed her children, and Child Protection Services might take them away. As a single mom, it kept her up at night. Together, we unpacked the worst-case scenario, which was that her car would break down unexpectedly. She asked herself the following question:

If the car breaks down one morning and I can't go to work, who can I call who will take me to work? She found out that her mom could come to pick up the children, and her best friend could take her to work. Both were able and willing to do that for about a week. After that, she would have to find another solution.

If the car could be fixed, how much could she afford to spend? At that time, she had no savings at all. All she could spare was about $100. Considering the value of the car, she decided that she would be ready to pay up to $1000 to fix it. Over that sum, she would buy another vehicle.

If the car couldn't be fixed, how much would she need to buy another one? After doing some research, she settled for $2500, as long as her dad could help her choose a reliable vehicle.

Just doing the research and seeing that there were options available to her eased her anxiety a bit. Even though she was still worried about her car breaking down, she realized that the chances of her running out of money altogether and not being able to care for her children were not rational. The second part of the plan was to prepare for the day when the car would break down. She acknowledged that if she had a system and was very intentional about it, she could most likely save $175 every week. If she started right away, she could pay to fix her car within about three months, and she could buy another vehicle if needed within eight to nine months. What had always seemed impossible was actually within reach. She had a plan, she started working on it, and her anxiety diminished drastically, especially at night.

Though eliminating the feelings of insecurity will be a substantial help, you also need to go further by creating a genuine sense of safety. Your next step will be to write a list of all the things that make you feel safe. They can be people, places, thoughts, songs, sounds, smells, and more. Sit down and ask yourself: "When do I feel the safest and the most serene?" Write down all the situations that come to mind and figure out how to recreate the same feeling of safety in your bedtime routine and your environment. You can bring items into your bedroom that contribute to your calmness. It could be a picture, a song, a sweater, a smell, anything that your mind associates with peace and tranquility and is not distracting or exciting. Isalou Regen, a French author, even suggests that you put together a "feel-good box" that contains all kinds of calming treasures to reassure you when you feel especially anxious.[42]

Most adults realize how important it is for children to create a sense of security when they go to bed. We make sure they have their favorite stuffed animal, their security blanket. We leave the door slightly open, and we keep a soft light on. We do these things to help them feel safe and fall asleep. As grown-ups, we forget that we, too, need to feel safe and that we need a certain ambiance to feel relaxed.

Write down below your list of serenity triggers and don't forget to update this list every time you experience a profound feeling of security and peace. Just like all the other worksheets in this book, the Serenity Triggers worksheet is part of the workbook that you can download and print for free at allonZcoaching.com/sleepitoff (use password SLEEP_IT_OFF).

List your serenity triggers below:

_____

_____

_____

_____

_____

_____

_____

_____

_____

When I launched my coaching practice, I had trouble sleeping for several months. A mix of both types of stress was involved: I was worried about finances, business plans, deadlines, and performance, among other things, but I was also excited to learn more, meet new people, exercise my passion, and see amazing results with my new clients. I just couldn't sleep at night because there was too much going on in my head, and no matter how tired I was, it was hard to unplug, and I always felt slightly on edge. One item that became part of my routine at that period was a tiny green notebook that I would always keep next to my bed in case I woke up in the middle of the night with the idea of the century. I don't wake up at night anymore, but knowing that the notebook is right there makes me feel safe. I know that if I come up with an idea during the night, I can write it down and go back to sleep immediately without forgetting it by the time I wake up the next day. This little notebook gives me peace of mind, even if I rarely use it.

14. I work on a computer all day and have to check emails at night.

As we have seen, blue light from screens affects our melatonin production. Darkness and low temperatures support melatonin production, whereas too much light exposure (especially blue light) will decrease production. Melatonin production is at its peak at around 3 or 4 am. If one wakes up around that time and exposes oneself to light, the process is disturbed, and it can be challenging to fall back to sleep.

To encourage melatonin production, our body needs to know the difference between day and night. If we stay indoors all day, working on a computer, and then are indoors at night, browsing the internet for fun, our body is not aware of the time of day and does not experience the increased melatonin release that occurs when we naturally transition from daylight to darkness. In such a situation, the light doesn't change as time goes on; it is just a steady light coming from screens and indoor lights. For our body to know the difference between waking hours and sleeping hours, we need to give it plenty of cues that will help differentiate day from night. Go outside, move, and get as much natural light as possible during the day. Slow down at night, dim the lights, and turn off your screens at least two hours before bedtime.

Some people use luminotherapy in the morning to make sure their body knows it is time to wake up. This can be helpful, especially if you suffer from seasonal depression. If you use luminotherapy (you can find lamps or glasses), make sure you do so as soon as you get up in the morning, during breakfast, for instance. Don't wait until the day is halfway through, or you will confuse your system even more. Some alarm clocks have a dawn simulator that starts before the alarm goes off so that your body gets the message that it will soon be time to wake up, even if it is still pitch-black outside.

Keep in mind that being outdoors as much as possible is the most critical step to take. You don't have to live in the countryside to be outside. You can find ways to increase your outdoor time without changing your schedule much and without needing recreational activities to do outside. For example, maybe you could walk places when you are running errands. You could sit by an open window, or sit in the yard or on the deck when you are making phone calls. Find all the ways you can be exposed to natural light. Not only will it show your body an apparent difference between day and night, but it might also increase your Vitamin D production.

15. I only sleep well when I am not at home.

If you struggle with sleep at home but have no problem when you are away, the first thing you need to do is check your environment for any disturbances that were mentioned previously. Are there blinking lights in your bedroom? Do you have blackout curtains? Is it quiet and cool at night? Are you staying alert because you don't know who might come in and disturb you? If you haven't done so yet, make sure you are changing your environment in a way that plays in your favor.

Another reason you sleep better when you are away from home might be a sense of responsibility and control. Many of us feel in charge when we are at home, and that is especially true for caregivers who stay alert all night in case a family member or a pet needs to be tended to. When we leave the house, either on vacation or on a work trip, we loosen up, let our guard down, and sleep better because we can relax. We might still be stressed out for different reasons, more tangible and easier to pinpoint. Still, the unconscious alertness is gone, and this is often enough to help our brain waves slow down.

So, if you sleep well when you are away from home, you must look at your responsibilities and your need for control or productivity when you are at home. Most people's sleep issues can't be fixed by buying a weighted blanket or special tea. Be ready to dig deep into your emotional needs to find ways to meet them without staying awake at night. Find out who you feel responsible for and how you might care for them in the long term while being well-rested. You might have to set new boundaries, share the burden with a reliable partner, or, more often than not, let go of your perfectionism.

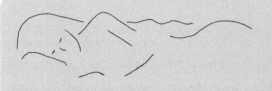

STORYTIME

When he came to see me, Nick had been struggling with his sleep for a few weeks, after separating from his girlfriend and her two children. It was a traumatic experience, and he missed the kids dearly. At night, Nick was agitated and his mind raced. He often could not fall asleep until early morning and was exhausted.

Nick had type 2 diabetes and was mostly interested in lowering his blood sugar levels and losing weight. That's why he came to health coaching. Sleep was not his top priority. He assumed that things would get back to normal after a while. As we worked together on increasing his level of physical activity and switching to a whole food diet, eating mostly plants and getting better at portion control, he started feeling more rested at night, but things were still far from ideal. Nick was anxious about bedtime, and the fear of not falling asleep grew bigger.

Nick was very busy at work but not overly stressed. He is a Project Manager in a start-up and is excellent at dealing with emergencies and making sure he doesn't get overwhelmed when crises arise. I made a mistake when coaching Nick. I assumed, for a few weeks, that working on task and time management was not necessary for him because he was a master in the field. But in fact, even though Nick excels at juggling multiple demanding projects at work, when it came to his personal life, prioritizing didn't come as naturally. He felt overwhelmed by his to-do list and had the feeling that he was always falling short and underachieving. The break-up reinforced this idea.

We decided that every week for a while, he would select one personal task or project to concentrate on for the whole week and would give himself permission to do nothing else from his to-do list that week. It was a challenging thought for an overachiever like Nick, but it worked right away. The first week, he decided to sort all his digital photos and back them up on an external drive. That was his project for the week; anything else would have to wait. The very first night, he slept 8 hours straight. The second night, same thing. It gave him confidence that he was onto something, and this allowed him to relax. The second week, he cleaned up his garage; after that, he pressure-washed his deck. He kept using the same strategy for a few weeks and went back to sleeping perfectly well. His fear of insomnia was gone. He would have been able to go back to tackling a few more projects at once, but he had realized that proceeding this way in his personal life was less stressful and he ended up keeping his "one-project-at-a-time routine" for as long as we worked together.

16. I only sleep well when I am at home.

Not being able to sleep well outside of our own home and bed is a widespread issue. For many people, it is not a problem because they spend most of their time at home rather than away. If you are not sleeping well when you are not in your typical environment, it is probably because you cannot recreate the safe haven you have at home. If it is a problem for you, try taking a picture of your usual sleeping environment and use this photo as a model for the room you are sleeping in while you are away. Do your best to reproduce your home sleeping environment by doing things such as blocking the light completely, using white noise to cover disturbances, etc.

For many, this problem might be due to the inability to feel safe outside of the home or to the inability to accept that we cannot be there for those who might need us at home.

For instance, a parent might monitor their phone throughout the night to make sure a spouse or children have not sent an SOS. If this is the case for you, take the time to find out whether or not you can trust the person who is in charge back home. If you can trust them, you need to work on disconnecting from your phone. You can also come to an agreement that people will only reach out to you if they have an emergency. Using the "do-not-disturb" function on your phone might be an excellent way to ensure that only critical calls will get through. Social media notifications and everything else can wait until the next day.

We often think that we are essential to other people's lives or our work. And we might be, to some extent. But most of the time, our family or business will do just fine if we are not available to them during the night. Realizing that you are not indispensable can be a hard thing to accept, but it can also dramatically lower your stress level.

Sleep is directly linked to the trust we have in people we love. Ask yourself whether trust might be the issue that keeps you from sleeping when you are away from your loved ones. If that's the case, you have some work to do.

17. I am on a low-carb diet and can't sleep.

I have met many people who were struggling with sleep while following a strict low-carb diet. It was difficult for them to understand that food was the issue. Some had been struggling with sleep long before starting the diet. Lack of physical activity, obesity, or type 2 diabetes were initially causing their sleep issues. After losing weight, they expected to sleep better. Unfortunately, that didn't happen because once they switched to a low-carb diet, their sleep issues had a new root.

As mentioned in situation #6, one explanation for this phenomenon is that carbohydrate intake leads to more serotonin production. Eating protein doesn't have the same effect on our hormone levels. This is why we often want to eat pasta, cookies, and sugary drinks when we feel stressed out, sad, or tired. Our brain knows that serotonin will make us feel better and pushes us to reach out for simple carbohydrates such as baked goods, processed foods, and sugar. The chief reason low-carb diets work for weight loss is that when we follow them, we cut out most processed foods. Processed foods account for the majority of calories consumed by most people. Keeping healthy, complex carbohydrates in our diet, such as vegetables, fruit, beans, and non-processed whole grain, is often a much healthier way to lose weight. It can also help you maintain a correct level of serotonin and, as a result, better sleep.[43]

18. I snooze for an hour each morning, and it is so hard to wake up.

Snoozing is a big no-no. It is a total waste of our time. We are not productive, yet we are not resting, either, since our sleep keeps being interrupted. Snoozing doesn't provide many benefits beyond instant gratification. The time we spend snoozing is very similar to the time we spend at night browsing our social media feed, not getting much out of it but also not being able to stop.

If you snooze 30 minutes every morning, you are depriving yourself of 30 minutes of sleep. Since you are not doing anything else, you are also wasting precious minutes that you could use in a more productive way, which would allow you to go to bed 30 minutes earlier at night. Whenever you snooze, you are losing both ways.

If you have been snoozing, my suggestion is that you stop right now. This is one of the rare straightforward recommendations I will give you. Instead of snoozing, decide at what time exactly you need to wake up, set your alarm, and put it far away from your bed so that you have to get up to turn it off. If you have been snoozing for 30 minutes for the past months or years, now is a great time to set your alarm to the early setting and use the extra time to do some exercise instead. It will get your body in motion, it will tell your brain that now is the time to wake up, and you will be able to squeeze in 10, 20 or 30 minutes of workout – high-intensity interval training (HIIT), stretching, yoga, whatever you like – without having to make extra room in your schedule since you were not doing anything during that time, anyway.

19. I wake up two or three times at night to use the restroom.

Many factors could make it hard to sleep through the night without using the restroom.

With age, many of us have trouble holding urine for as long as we used to. Getting up once at night to empty your bladder is not a big deal unless you can't fall back to sleep afterward. If that's your case, you might want to address your level of alertness after waking up rather than the need to urinate itself, which is quite normal.

When you go to the restroom, use a night-light in your hallway and bathroom so that you don't have to turn on the lights at all. If possible, consider going with your eyes mostly shut. Don't look at the time on your phone, don't check your messages, keep things as non-stimulating as possible, and avoid drinking a glass of water after using the restroom if it's hard for you to go back to sleep, as it signals to your body that it is time to wake up.

If you get up several times at night, you might also reconsider your fluid intake during the day. Sip small quantities of water throughout the day rather than gulping down a large glass with every meal, especially around dinner time. Increasing your water intake until about 4 pm and then not drinking after that time is also an option to consider, depending on your level of physical activity. Of course, I would also recommend that you get your blood sugar checked. One of the side effects of type 2 diabetes is an increased urge for emptying one's bladder. For someone who might have type 2 diabetes, it is critical to get diagnosed as soon as possible to take measures that will help control insulin and potentially reverse the disease or, at least, keep it from progressing.

The need to empty your bladder might not be the actual problem. Most of us, when we wake up in the morning, need to rush to the bathroom, yet we weren't woken up by this urge. As we have mentioned before, we can sleep through many minor disturbances, but it is when they add up that problems arise. If noise occurs or a light is blinking while your body needs to urinate and you are in a light sleep phase, chances are you will wake up. If your bedroom is utterly silent and dark, though, you might sleep through the physiological need. By the same token, if your bedroom is too warm or if you had a heavy meal and you start sweating while at the same time feeling the urge to go to the bathroom, you will wake up, because your brain can't handle these many perturbations without having you wake up.

Many factors can influence your sleep and your need to urinate, so you should consider all the disturbances involved and work your way through them to eliminate as many as possible.

20. It is hard to find the right temperature for a good night's sleep.

Your body is a brilliant machine. If your hands and feet are cold, your system will want to make sure that your core temperature doesn't drop as well, because that's where all the vital organs are.

When you go to bed, make sure your extremities are not cold; otherwise, your body will work hard to warm them up. As a result, your core temperature will rise and hinder the release of melatonin. Ideally, you want your feet and hands to be warmed up before you go to bed and while you sleep so that your core body temperature can drop as it should for melatonin production. To do so, you can take a warm bath or shower (not a hot one though, you don't want to raise your general body temperature), you can wear socks, mittens if your hands are too cold, and even a hat if needed (a great option if you go camping). Make sure also that you stay covered and comfortable and that the temperature of your bedroom stays between about 60 to 65 degrees Fahrenheit. Big fluffy down comforters are not always the best option, even if we love them because of the luxury. Getting a thinner down comforter might work best, and down tends to regulate temperature better than synthetic.

I live in Seattle, and the rule here is to dress in layers, no matter the time of the year. Dressing in layers for the night might be a good idea, especially if you wake up at night overheating and sweaty. For me, dressing in layers at night means wearing a tank top and a long-sleeve shirt when I first lie down. As the night goes on, I can take off the shirt and, if needed, the tank top too. My feet and hands are rarely cold at night, but in the wintertime, I often start the night with a scarf (short enough to avoid strangulation!).

If night sweats are an issue, you may also want to look into your food intake and see whether you are taking in too much food at the wrong time — or too many calories compared to the calories you burn throughout the day.

If you drink herbal tea before going to bed, make sure you are not drinking it too hot; otherwise, it will raise your body temperature and keep your body from releasing melatonin.

If you find it hard to wake up in the morning, make sure your hands and feet are not too warm, so that your body works on bringing your core temperature up a little and is ready for the day ahead.

21. My nighttime routine and rituals don't work.

Your routine is a sequence of actions you regularly follow without thinking much about them. For example, getting dressed, brushing your teeth, or going to work. Your routine consists of habits, whether healthy or unhealthy, and is pretty much unconscious. Rituals, as we have seen in chapter four, are more intentional than routine. You perform rituals mindfully and often with a specific purpose, such as relaxing or getting your mind and body ready for bed.

Your sleep routine should start in the morning. To help your body regulate itself and know when to wake up and when to fall asleep, it is helpful to have a cadence. A simple way to do this is to organize your days around regular meals at regular times.

- Eat a healthy breakfast, with protein and no added sugar, to tell your body that it is time to wake up and fuel for the day.
- Eat a well-balanced and reasonably portioned lunch to keep powering through the day.
- Eat a light dinner, including non-processed carbohydrates such as beans and whole grains, as well as vegetables, so that your body understands that night time is coming and activities are slowing down.

It might seem far-fetched that your breakfast will determine how well you sleep. Yet, the more consistency in your daily schedule, the easier it will be for your biological clock to regulate itself.

It is excellent to implement nighttime routines and rituals such as reading a book in bed and applying essential oil on your wrist. But if your schedule is all over the place for the rest of the day, it will be hard to convince your melatonin production gland that now is the time to go to sleep.

Give your body a heads-up at least one hour before bedtime. Set the alarm if necessary, and don't do any activity that is exciting or stressful or requires concentration after the alarm goes off. Instead, enjoy only relaxing activities and perform your rituals without doing anything that would lead your brain activity to pick up again.

As we have seen in chapter four, nighttime rituals can also help you feel less anxious because they provide your mind with a sense of security and peace, rather than the fear or excitement that a change between day and night might create.

Don't implement 15 rituals at once! Choose one or two rituals that are meaningful to you and be consistent with them. From washing your face and getting into comfortable pajamas, to reading a book while sipping herbal tea, or lighting a candle while listening to soft music and stretching, the sky is the limit when it comes to finding rituals that will help you prepare for sleep. When you pick a ritual, keep at it for a while before you decide that it doesn't work for you. Rituals are a brilliant way to calm your mind, make it feel safe, and allow the parasympathetic system to take over. But as long as they feel new to you, they might not work. It is once they are part of your routine that they will make you feel safe and help you transition into sleep.

22. I am too busy to sleep much during the week, but I catch up on weekends.

Unfortunately, you can't catch up on the weekend.

Let's compare sleep to a 401K for which your employer is matching contributions. When you save up to 5% of your salary, your employer will match your contributions. When you save 5%, it is like when you sleep all the hours you need. It is ideal because you are getting the maximum amount of free money from your employer, and you are also saving a lot.

If one month you save nothing, your employer won't match, so, you are losing money and can never make up that money because even if you contribute 10% the following month, your employer will only match 5%. It is still an excellent idea to save 10% because you will make up for what you have not set aside the month before. Still, the free money from your employer is lost forever.

It is the same with sleep. If you don't sleep enough during the week and then sleep two extra hours on the weekend, it will be good that you rest the extra time during the weekend because it will help you feel less sleep-deprived, but what you have missed out on during the week — growth hormones, leptin and ghrelin balance, better fat metabolism, etc. — is gone and you won't be able to get it back. Even if you sleep 10 hours on the weekend, you can't get back the hormones you have not produced during the week and other benefits of sleep.

23. I am exhausted after work and can't resist a nap.

This is a pretty common scenario. You have a tiring job, maybe because you work in construction, landscaping, or as a nurse in a hospital. When you come home after a long day, you are so exhausted that you don't even have the energy to fix and eat dinner. You go straight to your couch and take a nap. When you wake up two or three hours later, you are starving, order take out, and then can't fall back asleep until very late at night or even early in the morning. You might get the right amount of sleep, but it is not good-quality sleep and not at a time when your body would need it the most.

I don't often recommend that you stay up when you are tired, but in this situation, this is what I would suggest. If you are able to skip your nap, you might still be able to go to bed very early but could sleep through the night.

Consider taking a nap around lunchtime rather than when you come home from work. I have seen a lot of people nap in their car in a parking garage or alongside a park. A 30-minute nap in the middle of the day could be sufficient to help you stay awake long enough in the evening. Another option is to not come home right after work and instead run a few errands, go for a walk or to the gym, or meet up with friends. Of course, you are tired, but if you stay busy after work, you might be able to solicit enough energy to stay awake. If you are physically active, it will most likely help you have a better-quality sleep during the night, and if you stay outside and enjoy some daylight after work, your body will register that it is not yet time to sleep.

I also recommend that the night before, or the morning before you go to work, you plan for your dinner and make sure that when you get home at night, as much as possible is ready for you and you don't feel inclined to eat processed food or skip your meal altogether. If you can grab a nutritious dinner without having to prepare anything, you will be most likely to eat well and sleep well.

As always, if you feel that those changes are daunting, take your time. You can try this out two nights per week to start with. If it works, then you can expand to a few more days.

24. I go to bed late to avoid having sex

There can be many reasons why you are delaying your bedtime with the hopes that when you hit the pillow, your partner will be sound asleep and won't want to engage in sex. For some people, lack of libido is the reason why they want to avoid intimacy. For others, it is trauma, chronic pain, or a poor body image. I have had a client who was worried about having a heart attack. Whatever the reason, one thing most people have in common is that they feel very guilty about their lack of sex drive or their incapacity to fulfill their partner's desire and most of them don't open up easily about the issue.

If that is your case, it is critical to turn this seemingly personal problem into a challenge that you address head-on with your partner, as a team. Indeed, you are both suffering the consequences, and if you keep going to bed past your bedtime, there is very little chance that things will ever get better since you will most likely add fatigue and irritability to the root cause of the problem.

I am not going to walk you through a conversation with your partner. I am not a counselor and it is not the topic of this book. But I would like to offer two simple options to help you take the very first step, which is to go back to your natural sleep schedule rather than delaying your bedtime. Indeed, if you are not sleeping as much as you need to, chances are it will be hard to solve the problem, even if your partner is on board.

The first option is for you to temporarily sleep away from your partner, until you "catch up" on sleep. Doing so for a week or two will allow you to get a full night's sleep without feeling any pressure for sex. You will be able to bring your body back to its natural rhythm, and once you feel refreshed and rested again, then you can start looking for a long-term solution as a couple.

The second option is to make a deal with your partner and commit to not have sex at all for an entire week or maybe two weeks if that's what you need to feel rested again. On top of letting you sleep as much as you need, you might be surprised by the effect that such a pause might have on your relationship. Again, the goal here is for you to get enough sleep without feeling pressured or guilty. Explaining the purpose to your partner is very important to avoid them feeling rejected. Furthermore, having a deadline is reassuring for everybody.

Those two options are only for the first step. You will need to address the problem at its root after that, but if you don't rest first, you might not be in the best disposition and could damage your relationship.

25. I have been sleep-deprived for too long; I always will be.

The first time a client mentioned this to me, I was surprised because I had never thought about it this way. This client had a newborn, and because she had read that you could not catch up on sleep, she was terrified that she would never feel rested again in her life. Her logic made complete sense. Fortunately, that is not true. She was correct that the benefits she had missed out on while not sleeping enough were gone forever. Still, it didn't mean that she would never feel perfectly rested again.

We have just compared sleep to a 401K savings account. Now let's compare sleep to your vacation days. Imagine that you get ten days per year, and every January, the clock resets to zero, whether or not you use your vacation days. If you don't take a vacation one year, what is lost is lost. You will never make up for the trip you have missed and for the memories you have not created. Yet, if you have never taken your 10 days of vacation so far and you start taking them every year from now on, you will experience great things, relax, create new memories, discover new places, and enjoy all the amazing benefits of a long vacation. You won't make up for the lost time, but you will still have a marvelous time going forward.

The same goes for sleep. The hours you have not slept are gone. You can't get them back. But it is never too late to do the right thing, and you will most likely experience the benefits quickly once you start sleeping enough.

• • •

Hopefully, you found answers and ideas browsing through those real-life situations. We are all unique, though, so, most likely, your story didn't fit perfectly well into one situation. Still, you might have gotten some suggestions that you can tweak slightly, just as you would tweak a template.

If you are still at a loss, I encourage you to contact me through my website allonZcoaching.com so that we can brainstorm together. Sometimes, it doesn't take much to figure out potential steps forward. I have found that talking with someone who doesn't belong to your life can help you think outside the box, especially when they have a slightly different cultural background and some expertise in the field.

Now, some special situations don't fit in the mold. From menopause to night shift work, from jet lag to napping, let's review some of them in the next chapter.

CHAPTER EIGHT
Special Focus On...

The issues addressed in this chapter affect only a small number of people, but they are also tough to tackle and require particular attention. In the following pages, we will look in more detail at:

- Menopause
- Naps
- Night and shift work
- Jetlag when traveling to a different time zone
- Night terrors in children

MENOPAUSE

Though menopause comes with many symptoms, poor sleep is one of the most commonly experienced ones. Whether they have issues falling asleep, wake up frequently during the night, or can't sleep in despite being exhausted, 39 to 47% of perimenopausal women, and 35 to 60% of postmenopausal women deal with insomnia.[1]

Common reasons for poor sleep around menopause include depression, anxiety, hot flashes, snoring, and sleep apnea. According to Grace Pien, M.D., M.S.C.E., an assistant professor of medicine at the Johns Hopkins Sleep Disorders Center, "Postmenopausal women are two to three times more likely to have sleep apnea compared with premenopausal women."[2]

If you believe that sleep apnea is a problem for you, refer to chapter five to find out more about the causes of sleep apnea and what you can do about them. If you are struggling with depression and anxiety as you go through menopause, you will also have to address the root of the problem, and I encourage you to talk to your health care provider to see whether counseling or hormone replacement therapy could be an option. Don't cross your fingers, hoping that things will improve on their own. They might, but they might also get worse, and no one deserves to be miserable for years when there are solutions available to you.

Hot flashes affect 75 to 85% of women going through menopause. They are defined as "unexpected feelings of heat all over the body accompanied by sweating." They often concentrate around the face and the chest, and even though they don't last very long (a few minutes), they are very disruptive because they usually lead to awakening. If we were to wake up for two to three minutes and go back to sleep right away, hot flashes might not be such a problem. But often, we become frustrated, our mind starts racing, we need to go to the bathroom, and a three-minute hot flash turns into a two-hour-long lapse in our sleep. A lot of women end up exhausted and also become apprehensive even before going to sleep because they fear that they will wake up and not be able to fall back to sleep. More about this vicious cycle in chapter five.[3]

Hot flashes are linked to hormonal changes. But even without taking hormone treatments, there are steps you can take to reduce the occurrence and severity of hot flashes and also limit the impact they will have on your sleep.

- Just as you would work on treating depression and anxiety at their root, it is essential to eliminate as many sources of stress as possible from your life. Also, learn "on-the-spot" stress reduction strategies such as meditation, cardiac coherence breathing, and self-hypnosis so that you can fall back asleep relatively quickly after a hot flash episode. You can refer to situations #10 and #12 in chapter seven for stress relief techniques. Also, can we add internal links back to those situations?
- Make sure that your sleeping environment is cool and comfortable and that you are not overheating in your bedroom and between your sheets. Dress in layers, not only during the day but also at night so you can shed clothes easily when you get too hot. As mentioned in situation #20 in chapter seven, I usually go to bed with a tank top and a long-sleeved shirt. After reading for a while, I feel warm enough to take off the shirt but always keep it handy in case it gets chilly. If, on the contrary, I feel too hot for some reason, I still have the tank top that I can remove.
- Make sure your dinner is light and doesn't contain red meat or fried food. Try to stop eating before you are full and at least two or three hours before going to bed.
- Avoid foods, beverages, and substances that do not promote sleep: caffeine, chocolate, caffeinated tea, alcohol, cannabis, nicotine, etc.

- Spicy foods can also increase hot flashes. Soy-based foods might help reduce hot flashes because "among postmenopausal women, soy may act more like an estrogen."[4] Adding soy into your diet in a reasonable amount might bring some relief. It is essential to know that soy might have side effects, though, so talk to your doctor first, especially if you have a history of breast cancer.[5]

- Focusing on dinner might not be enough. You might have to give up certain foods altogether and also reduce your food intake during the day. As mentioned in chapter five, most of us need to eat less if we want to sleep better. This is especially relevant if you suffer from hot flashes.

NAPS

Naps are a great way to recover if you have a bad night or when you go through a phase in life when you cannot sleep as much as you need, for instance, when you have a newborn, experience the loss of a loved one, or go through a transition in life such as a divorce or layoff.

Shawn Stevenson, author and creator of The Model Health Show, used the following analogy, in one of his podcasts, to describe naps and how we can use them: If we were to compare sleep to food, we could say that sleeping at night is like eating real, nutritious foods, and taking naps is like taking supplements.[6] Unfortunately, many people rely on supplements to get all the nutrients they need for their body to function well, but it is far from ideal. Naps, just like supplements, should be used to compensate for deficiencies or, with sleep, to mitigate temporary sleep deprivation. Naps will help, but there are benefits from a good night's sleep that you won't get through a nap, just like there are many benefits from eating real food that you can't get from eating supplements because supplements cannot bring such a large variety of nutrients as real whole foods can. Among other things, a short nap after lunch won't help you reach the perfect balance between your different appetite hormones (ghrelin and leptin) the way a good night's sleep will.

Naps, even though they might not help with hormones and some other aspects of our sleep, can help us feel fresh again and regenerated during the day. They can sometimes be a life-saver!

It is true that a nap can ruin your sleep at night, but it is not always the case. If you love, or if you need, to take naps – both being excellent reasons – you will have to monitor the effects it has or doesn't have on the quality of your sleep at night. For most people, taking naps later in the afternoon will keep them up at night, but for others, it might just shift their sleep schedule. There is a good chance that taking a 20- or 30-minute nap around lunchtime won't do you much harm. It is crucial to experiment, though, because it is your sleep, your body, and you are unique.

If your naps are too long and you accidentally drift into a deep sleep phase, not only will you wake up very groggy (by an alarm or a disruptive sound), but you might also use up some of your "accrued tiredness" (chapter four), which will keep you from falling asleep later at night.

Our body is wired to slow down at midday. About six hours after we get up, chances are we will experience a need to sleep. We often think that this dip occurs because we ate lunch. It could well be if we ate processed carbs and other sweet or fatty foods. Still, it can also be because our internal clock lowers our cortisol level, and our blood pressure drops slightly at that time of the day, a perfectly normal phenomenon (National Sleep Foundation 2018).[7]

It is recommended to favor "power naps" if possible. Power naps are very short (about 10 to 20 minutes) and will help us feel relaxed, refreshed, and regenerated without allowing us into a deep sleep phase. Most of us have noticed that sometimes, we barely fall asleep and just drift away for a few minutes, yet feel much better than before when our brain kicks in again.

NIGHT AND SHIFT WORK

If you are working night shifts and struggling with sleep, you are not alone. In 2018, almost 20% of European Union workers were working nights, compared to about 10% in the early years of the century.[8]

According to 2004 data from the Bureau of Labor Statistics, "Almost 15 million Americans work full time on evening shift, night shift, rotating shifts, or other employer-arranged irregular schedules."[9]

But what exactly is shift work? A shift worker is anyone who works outside the typical "nine to five" schedule. Whether you are a nurse working at the hospital three nights per week, a grocery store employee shelving product from 9 pm to 4 am, or anyone else who works while the rest of us are sleeping, you have an extra challenge to deal with. Here are some tips and recommendations on what you can try to make your sleep healthier and more regenerating.

Like many others in your situation, you probably find it hard to balance sleep and daily activities with your work schedule, especially if this schedule is unreliable and inconsistent. We have talked extensively about the fact that the general population rarely prioritizes sleep. With the challenges faced by night and shift workers, it makes it even harder to get enough quality sleep.

If you work shifts, there are three key reasons why you might suffer from sleep deprivation.

- Your biological clock is set up to sleep during the night, not during the day, so you are always going against your body's natural needs.
- The external cues that help your body establish a robust sleep schedule are not available when you are trying to sleep: it is bright outside and noisy, etc. On the opposite end, at night, your body receives signals that it should relax: it is dark, the environment might be quieter, etc. Yet that's the time when you go to work and need to be productive, sharp, and alert.
- Our society is set up to accommodate people who work during the day. It is harder for you to find time to sleep, especially since people around you might expect you to be up and running all day even though you have also worked all night. Not only do you have to be extremely disciplined to sleep as much as your body needs, but you also have to justify to others why you sleep when everyone else is up.

Sleep deprivation is not the only consequence of shift work. Because it is so hard to establish a regular sleep pattern, many night workers will end up also living their daily life more chaotically: irregular meal schedules, snacking, lack of consistency with exercise programs, higher consumption of caffeine and tobacco, and more.

There are a few steps you can take to prevent sleep deprivation and negative repercussions on your health.

- Prioritize your sleep. It is even more important for you than for the people around you because *your* environment will always work against you.
- Keep your schedule as regular as possible. It will help your body know what to expect regarding sleep and food intake.
- Adopt healthy eating habits so that your level of energy is at its peak, your immune system is optimized, and your body can recover fast from anything that is thrown your way.

Tips to Feel Better During Your Shift

- Take breaks during your shift, if you can, and fit a 20- to 30-minute catnap. If sleeping is not an option at work, try to at least take short and regular breaks and use them to breathe, get some fresh air, stretch, and move around.

- Drink water regularly and make sure you are never dehydrated. Bring a bottle of water to work and make sure you finish it while on the job. If you need reminders, set up alarms on your phone. For the first few months, you might need external reminders to drink water. Still, after a while, your body will become accustomed to your habits. You will feel thirsty more naturally.

- Expose yourself to light as much as possible just before and during your work shift. Ideally, take a walk outside while it is still bright and just before going to work, to signal to your body that it is time to be up and alert.

- Eat a warm, nutritious, and healthy meal during work hours and avoid snacking throughout your shift or once you are at home. Try to keep your eating schedule regular and consistent throughout the week.

- Be physically active during the day, when you are not working, and especially right before your shift. Make sure to balance the need for exercising with the need for sleep, though, and prioritize sleep when you don't have time to do both. For example, if you have a 30-minute window right before work, and you have found no other time to sleep, taking a nap may be more beneficial than going on a quick jog.

Tips to Get Better Sleep

- Avoid consuming caffeinated beverages, except maybe right before your shift. Otherwise, caffeine might keep you from falling asleep or from sleeping well after work.

- Expose yourself to darkness right after your shift, and if possible, go to bed straight after work. If you finish working in the morning, and it is already bright outside, think about wearing sunglasses on the way home from work to keep your brain from registering the daylight. Keeping your body in the dark will encourage melatonin production.

- Break up your sleep if needed: sleeping eight hours at once might be out of reach, but you can still get to eight hours by sleeping one, two, or three times during the day for shorter periods. Research has shown that during the day, our sleep is more restful before 10 am or 11 am, and then again between 1 pm and 5 pm. To feel more refreshed and rested, you can try to get used to a regular two-shift sleeping schedule. Go to bed as soon as possible when getting home from work and sleep until about 10 or 11 am. Go back to bed for a few hours between 1 pm and 5 pm after having taken care of your daily chores. By using this method, you have higher chances of reaching enough hours of sleep per day, and you will end up with a deeper and more regenerating sleep, which is critical. Establishing a relatively regular schedule for your primary sleep time and your naps is ideal as it will allow your body to adjust to those times, which will make it easier for you to fall asleep and wake up when you need to.

- Include physical activity in your day once you have your sleep needs covered.
- Be organized and plan your activities in advance to mitigate the need to react to life's unpredictable events. This will minimize the number of last-minute and flaw-prone decisions you will have to make regarding food and sleep.

As always, don't implement all these strategies and new routines at once. Concentrate on one or two habits that you want to work on and take your time. For example, reduce snacking little by little, bring a warm lunch to work two times per week, or get your loved ones involved to support you. It is imperative to start small and progress steadily rather than rushing through the process.

JET LAG

Adjusting to different time zones is tough for most people. When traveling for vacation, you might not suffer as much because you can sleep in and nap and don't need as much brainpower. You can even go to bed whenever you feel like it. But when you are traveling for work and have to get up for meetings, present at conferences, and be at your best while feeling groggy, the whole experience turns into a nightmare. Not to mention traveling with little ones, who might be jet-lagged too, but for some reason, are on a completely different schedule than yours. They can turn into real monsters!

Let's go over the reasons why traveling to another time zone can be so hard on our system and how we can mitigate its effects.

Traveling to the West

When you travel to the West, you end up in a zone that is behind you time-wise, and you will have to wait longer before you can go to bed. As we have mentioned before, this is something our body can do relatively easily. We can postpone bedtime and accumulate more fatigue with little effort. In the morning, our biological clock will want us to wake up early, but since we will have spent several hours sleeping, we won't feel too bad waking up earlier in this time zone. Little by little, thanks to external light, our body will adjust. Usually, it takes about one day per hour of time difference.

To help your body adjust, you can try to spend as much time as possible outdoors, and make sure you expose yourself to daylight as much as possible in the afternoon and evening, so that your body knows it is not yet time to go to bed.

When traveling to the West, try to go to bed as early as socially reasonable and personally acceptable. This way, you will get as much sleep as you can before your biological clock wakes you up very early. You will adjust to the new time zone without being exhausted, stressed, and grumpy. It will also be easier to come home and adjust back to your previous time because you won't be as tired, and your biological clock won't be too disturbed. If you try to go to bed as late as possible, chances are you will still wake up very early the next day and will end up really sleep-deprived.

Traveling to the East

Traveling to the East is trickier because you get to a time zone where you have to go to bed before your body is ready to sleep. When your biological clock is telling you that it is not yet night time, and you lie in bed trying to sleep, you get agitated, frustrated, and nervous. Falling asleep becomes even harder. Depending on the length of your flight, the first night might go well, especially if you have skipped an entire night of sleep while in transit. In this case, you have accumulated such an enormous sleep debt that even though your melatonin production is low, you will crash and sleep just fine. But after that first night, sleeping may become challenging, and staying awake during the day could be a nightmare.

To help you adjust, it is crucial to spend as much time outdoors as possible, especially in the morning, to inform your body that it is time to wake up. You also want to stop using any kind of phone or laptop screen long before bedtime and try to reproduce your usual bedtime routine, so that your body and brain can pick up on the regular cues to sleep.

Tips for All Travelers

Whether you travel east or west, there are a few strategies to keep in mind.

- Don't be sleep-deprived before you travel. Sleep deprivation never helps. When traveling, it is not the accumulation of fatigue — or lack of accumulation — that keeps you from sleeping. It is your biological clock not being in phase with the actual time zone you arrive in. If you want to sleep better, you need to work on the biological clock. Being sleep-deprived will only add to the problem because you will be stressed out and agitated and will most likely make poor eating choices, which never helps. Try to be as rested as possible before you travel. Your body, your nervous system, and your emotional system will be much more resilient. Plus, we all know that planes are full of germs, so if you are tired, you are at a higher risk of catching a cold.

- If you travel overnight, try to sleep on the plane. Again, this will help you arrive relatively well-rested. Bring earplugs, an eye mask, comfortable clothes, and a light blanket. Most airlines bring the temperature down dramatically during the night, so make sure you have warm socks, a sweater, and a scarf. Even if you are not planning on sleeping on the plane, take earplugs and an eye mask on every trip, to use in hotel rooms. You never know when they are going to put you next to the elevator or on a floor with a party crowd!

- If you are traveling with children, don't skip their nap that day, hoping it will help them sleep on the plane. We all know that a tired baby is a cranky baby. It is not a good idea to keep a child from sleeping. What you can do on the day of travel and on the plane is keep your child away from any form of sugar, including juice, candy bars, chocolate, sweetened yogurt or applesauce, and any kind of processed food. The best way to keep a child from being agitated is to feed them whole foods instead of processed treats and snacks. Of course, this is something they need to be used to ahead of time, otherwise, they will be even more cranky.

- Avoid coffee, tea, and alcohol on the plane as much as you can – unless liquor is the only way for you to not strangle your travel partner out of pure fear of flying. Do what you can with what you have; find what works best for you. Just remember that caffeine can still have strong stimulating effects for up to nine or ten hours.[10] We have talked extensively about alcohol already. You can refer back to chapter five if you have been sleeping through that part of the book. While you limit beverages that will make you dehydrated and most likely agitated, it is always a good idea to increase your water intake before, during, and after a flight.

- A few days before you fly, start adjusting to the time zone you are traveling to by getting up early if you're traveling to the East or sleeping in at home if you're traveling to the West. For international trips, it can help you feel more human when you get there!

NIGHT TERRORS

Though night terrors can be a problem for anyone, it is mostly children who are affected. However, the effects usually ripple through the entire family.

Night terrors affect almost 40% of children, and even though they are very distressing, they are not usually a cause for concern. They typically happen during the first part of the night, when deep sleep is the most important. When subject to a night terror, a child will sit up terrified and sweaty, and usually screaming. There is not much you can do, as a parent, during the crisis itself. Your child will be very hard to wake up and will seem inconsolable. The good news is that most of the time, children won't remember the episode and aren't affected by night terrors unless they become so frequent that the child ends up sleep-deprived.

Even though we have little power during a night terror to help our child, besides keeping them safe in case they become very agitated or start sleepwalking, there are some factors that promote sleep terrors which parents can influence.

Tired and Cranky Children

Night terrors are aggravated by exhaustion and sleep deprivation. When a kid is exhausted because they stayed awake for too long, the chance that they will experience night terrors goes up. Therefore, night terrors can begin when a child is just starting to forgo nap time during the day. It is thus imperative to make sure your children are getting enough sleep and taking naps when needed. As parents, we have all noticed how cranky our little ones become when they transition out of napping. If your children are suffering from night terrors, maybe the transition was premature and you could go back to their previous schedule. Napping can be difficult for some children, so establishing a routine with a very regular schedule is essential. If your child is too awake to sleep, try going for a drive or a stroller ride in the neighborhood right before nap time. If your child is at a time in their life when they can't nap anymore, consider changing their schedule so they get the same amount of sleep they used to get when they napped; let them sleep a little longer and put them to bed a little earlier.

Sometimes, we believe that keeping our child from sleeping too much will help improve the quality of their sleep, so we postpone bedtime, we cut naps short, and we don't let them sleep in. Unfortunately, these measures often make the problem even worse.

A well-rested child is at lower risk for night terrors than a tired one.

Make sure your children are not:
- Getting up too early because they want to be on their tablet while you are sleeping in or getting ready;
- Going to bed too late because the family routine is organized in such a way that they have to stay up late;

- Giving up their naps prematurely because they want to or because it is more convenient for the family;
- Sleep-deprived. Assuming that your child might not be getting the rest they need is an excellent way to approach night terrors.

Stress

Stress will also make night terrors more frequent. We don't always realize the stress involved in our little ones' lives, yet it can be intense and will affect the quality of their sleep.

Having to rush from one activity to another, not having time to relax and feel lazy, being overwhelmed by requests, solicitations, and expectations, and being exposed to technology throughout the day can generate stress. We might not see screens as a source of tension since our children are watching cute shows and educational programs, but screens are not promoting relaxation. They keep children in a state of alertness that can become stressful.

It is essential to look at what stresses us out as adults and try to see how those stressors affect our children too. It is difficult – and not desirable – to shield our children from all sources of stress. Still, it is worth eliminating as many unnecessary sources of stress as possible from their lives, especially chronic stress.

Disrupted Sleeping Schedule

If your child is prone to night terrors, any change in their sleep pattern might exacerbate the problem. Traveling, house guests, holidays, illness, and giving up a nap are all examples of changes in their sleeping patterns. We cannot always keep our kids on a perfectly planned schedule, and it is fine to break the routine once in a while, but try to keep disruptions occasional. A child who does not have a sleep routine will be more affected by night terrors than a child who goes to bed and wakes up at regular times.

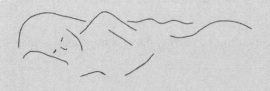

STORYTIME

Jenn is a perfectionist. She is a full-time mom and wife. Everything she does, she does amazingly well. She is a planner, she makes sure everything runs smoothly, she organizes the best parties and the best vacations. She volunteers at the Food Bank and the local library. Her life seems perfect, and Jenn is happy and fulfilled. When her twin boys start school, she will go back to work. She has it all figured out.

But when I started working with Jenn, she was exhausted and felt extremely guilty for falling asleep on the couch several times per week after lunch. It was challenging for her to let go and relax. She felt responsible for everything that was happening in her house, whether at night or during the day, whether she was alone with the kids or together with her husband. She woke up every two or three hours and would check on the boys, check on the dog, check on the door, or even check her phone to make sure her parents had not called.

The only way for Jenn to not feel in charge was to remove herself from her environment. She took the tough decision to go sleep at her mother's two nights per week. Twice a week, she would not be in charge. Twice a week, she would not be able to help. Twice a week, she would sleep 9 hours straight and wake up perfectly rested. Her husband and children survived just fine, and she caught up on some highly needed sleep.

Jenn got in touch with me one year after we had stopped working together. She reported that her decision to sleep at her mom's had utterly changed her life and her family's. The kids got a chance to bond with their father and expect more from him when they were in need. The dad himself realized everything he could give to his children, and it provided him an incentive and the needed self-confidence to become more involved in his children's lives. For Jenn, it was like a deliverance. She realized that she could be an amazing mom without micro-managing and controlling everything and that she could give herself permission to not be involved 24/7.

Sharing the Load

Whether or not our children experience night terrors, having young children often leads to decreased sleep in our lives as parents. Dopamine in our brain will keep us alert during the night and make sure we wake up if a disturbance in our environment is perceived. Initially, it kept us safe from predators. Now, it mostly allows us to keep our children safe, happy, and comfortable. The result of this selective attention is that we might not hear the garbage truck outside our window, but the slightest complaint from our baby will make us jump.

When there are two parents involved, it might be an excellent idea to take turns being responsible for the kids at night. If we do this, it is critical that we trust our partner 100% and completely release control; otherwise, it won't work. Take time before bed to discuss what the other caregiver will do if your child needs something, and take extra time on your own to convince yourself that you are not in charge that night. Otherwise, you will wake up at the slightest cry, and instead of one sleep-deprived parent, there will be two. Accept the fact that the other parent might not deal with night disturbances the way you do. They might let the baby cry longer than you would. They might give them a cold bottle instead of a warm one. They might forget to change a diaper. But you need to let go, and when it is their turn to take care of the baby, as long as no one is in danger, let them handle it their way and don't get involved. Remember, you are not as indispensable as you think you are. Use wax earplugs if that helps, and sleep as far away as possible if necessary.

• • •

If after reading this book, completing the worksheets, and making changes in your lifestyle you still haven't been able to find answers to your sleep problems, though, it might be time to turn to a more medicalized approach. Even though there is no way around them, lifestyle changes are not always sufficient, and you might require help from a specialist to identify sleeping aids that could be safe and effective for you.

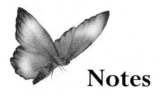

Notes

CHAPTER NINE
Time to Get Help?

Sleep is a puzzle, and it often takes time and effort to assemble all the pieces. Good sleep starts with a healthy lifestyle and a lot of self-awareness. Changing the way we eat, drink, move, and feel during the day often changes the way we sleep. For some, though, active days, good sleep hygiene, healthy eating, or night rituals are not enough. They need more, and despite their best attempts, they cannot do it on their own. They need to reach out for help.

Once you have worked hard to improve your sleep with behavioral changes and by taking into consideration all the aspects of your life, seeing a doctor and talking about the next step might be necessary. If your attempts have been unsuccessful, a health care provider might refer you to a sleep specialist who will help you identify the root of the problem and might prescribe medication or supplements.

NUTRIENT DEFICIENCY

Running some blood work is often a good idea. Our sleep can be affected by certain deficiencies in vitamins or minerals. Talking with a naturopath or another health care provider to find out whether you might have a nutrient deficiency is an easy step to take.

Vitamin D

Vitamin D deficiency can interfere with good sleep. Even if you have a very healthy diet, rich in salmon and other fatty fish such as tuna and mackerel, and even if you eat beef liver regularly (don't you?), you might still be vitamin D deficient depending on where you live and your exposure to sunlight. Indeed, most of the vitamin D we store comes from the sun.

Magnesium

Magnesium helps with sleep in many different ways. Among other things:

- Magnesium is a depressant,[1] which means that it helps you relax. Magnesium helps with stress reduction by acting directly in parts of the brain that regulate the stress hormone adrenaline, also known as epinephrine.[2]
- Magnesium also affects serotonin production. It is been shown that magnesium deficiency in the brain leads to lower levels of serotonin, the precursor for melatonin production.[3] Lack of serotonin can also be involved in depression, one of the numerous factors that may lead to insomnia.
- Magnesium deficiency may also lead to cramps, which often cause people to wake up in the middle of the night.[4]

If you want to make sure plenty of magnesium makes it to your plate every day, eat foods that are rich in fiber: green leafy vegetables (spinach, chard, kale, collard greens), legumes (lentils, beans, garbanzo beans), nuts, seeds, and non-processed whole grains.[5] Avocados and dark chocolate are also good sources of magnesium.

Magnesium can also be absorbed by the skin, using a spray right on your legs where they are cramping. An Epsom salts bath is also good for magnesium absorption, which makes a nighttime bath a winning go-to ritual for many. Calcium deficiency might also cause cramps, so make sure you get blood work done if you have cramps, and don't dismiss dehydration as a culprit for cramping.

Nutrient deficiency cannot always be solved with healthy food intake. If you are deficient, a medical provider can recommend appropriate supplementation.

> **DID YOU KNOW?**
> If your eyelids are twitching randomly, that might also be an indication that you are magnesium deficient.[6]

SUPPLEMENTS

Supplements can be safe and effective, but they can also be hazardous or useless. Only take supplements after talking with a healthcare provider and handle them the way you would handle prescription drugs. Just because supplements might be labeled "natural? doesn't make them safe.

Scary Facts about Supplements

- **Supplements can interact with other supplements or medication.**

Don't take them thinking they are unconditionally safe. That is not true, and even though an herbal supplement seems harmless, you need to know that natural medicine is powerful and, as a result, should not be treated lightly.

- **Supplements are not well regulated in the United States.**

In the United States, when it comes to supplements, regulations look only at the quality of production: whether employees wash their hands when making the supplement, whether the bottle is made out of non-toxic material, that kind of thing. These considerations are essential, of course, but they have nothing to do with supplement safety or efficiency. It is up to the manufacturer to assess whether or not their product is safe or effective. The Food and Drug Administration (FDA) cannot get involved until problems are reported, which is *after* the supplement has been sold and consumers have experienced issues or complications. There might be plenty of unsafe supplements in the aisles of your grocery store, and by the time they are banned from the shelves, you might already have used them. I encourage you to learn more on the FDA website under food/dietary supplements.[7]

- **Not all brands are alike when it comes to the quality of supplements.**

What's on the label of a supplement is not necessarily what's in the bottle. A study conducted by the University of Ontario found that some sleeping supplements had far less of the active ingredient than was written on the label – which is not dangerous but decreased their effectiveness – while others had over 400% more of the active ingredient than what was advertised on the label. If someone thought they were taking 100 mg of melatonin, for instance, they were actually taking 400 mg. Considering that taking too much melatonin can mess up your ability to sleep, as we will see a bit later, this is frightening information.[8] The study also reported that some supplements contained active ingredients that were not present on the label.

If taking supplements is an option you are considering, check out the ConsumerLab website. It is a website referencing supplements that have been third-party tested. It can be a great way to make sure that what you are buying is of good quality and contains active ingredients as labeled. For instance, a product review by ConsumerLab of 17 valerian supplements revealed that four did not contain valerian at all, four had half the amount listed, two were contaminated by lead, and one was contaminated by cadmium.[9]

Side Effects

There are plenty of supplements that might be suggested to help you sleep better and especially alleviate anxiety and stress. My approach is based on behavioral changes rather than supplementation, and I don't have the expertise or authority to recommend supplements. If you decide to use supplements, though, I would like to draw your attention to the fact that even common herbal treatments like lavender, lemon balm, valerian, passionflower or kava can lead to side effects such as liver damage, drowsiness, confusion, headaches, low blood pressure, increased appetite, abdominal pain and more. Even chamomile can increase the risk of bleeding when used with blood-thinning drugs. Furthermore, the efficiency of these herbal remedies might not be proven.[10]

Again, handle supplements the way you would handle medicine. Talk to your health care provider for guidance and expert advice.

Melatonin

As a supplement, melatonin is often referred to as the magic pill for sleeping problems because it supposedly has no side effects. Melatonin might not have the usual side effects that sleeping pills have (hangover, physical addiction, and more). Still, it can have side effects such as headache, drowsiness, and nausea, and, most importantly, if you take too much of it, it can wreak havoc on your sleep in the long run.

As we have seen before, melatonin is a hormone that our body produces naturally. To understand how our body regulates melatonin production, think of the temperature in your home. Imagine the thermostat is in the living room, and you have a fireplace there too. When you make a fire, the temperature in the living room will rise. The thermostat will register the higher temperature and turn the furnace off, even though there is most likely not enough heat produced from the fireplace to keep the rest of the house at a comfortable temperature. If you keep a fire in the living room at all times, your furnace won't turn on very often and will become rusty and nonfunctional from disuse. If your fire dies, your boiler will no longer function, and your house will be cold.

Melatonin regulation works in a similar way. If you always give your body melatonin through supplementation, it might result in your production of melatonin decreasing. Furthermore, according to Professor Richard Wurtman, Director of MIT's Clinical Research Center, when the melatonin receptors in the brain are exposed to too much melatonin, they can become unresponsive.[11] If you take too much melatonin – for instance, because the label on your bottle gives you the wrong information – it might become harder to sleep in the long term.

Most of us produce melatonin naturally. When we take melatonin supplements, we are just adding melatonin to our natural production. But melatonin is only one of the five requirements for sleep. It will help with the timing of your biological clock, which is why melatonin can be a great temporary solution when you are jet-lagged. Melatonin tells your body and brain that you are tired and will make you ready for sleep even though you might not feel sleepy because of the time difference.

But if you are stressed out, had a big meal before bed, or sleep in a bedroom with blinking lights and a snoring dog, melatonin supplements won't make much of a difference. Melatonin, whether you take it as a supplement or not, does not make you sleep. It prepares your body for sleep, and once you are asleep, it ensures that your rest is of good quality. But even if you take melatonin supplements or produce enough melatonin on your own, you still have to do the work to make sure everything else sets you up for success.

As we have said before, darkness is a trigger for melatonin increase in the body, and melatonin production is at its peak around 3 am. Light in general and blue light, in particular, diminish our production of melatonin. So, if you take your tablet, phone, or laptop to bed, chances are you won't be able to produce as much melatonin as needed to fall asleep. Removing screens and the blue light they emit from our bedroom and our lives at least a couple of hours before bedtime is one of the simplest steps – unfortunately, not the easiest – we can take to make sure our melatonin production is sufficient, and we won't need supplementation.

With melatonin, just as with other supplements, be cautious and make sure you are following your doctor's recommendations. Whatever supplement you might be considering, it is vital never to assume that it is safe and without consequences. Talk to a health care provider and follow instructions. And as always, remember that there is no magic pill. If your lifestyle doesn't change, you won't experience lasting results.[12]

SLEEPING MEDICATION

Sleeping pills are not necessarily all evil. They are what they are – drugs – and sometimes, we need them. If you need sleeping pills, there is no need to feel bad about it or consider it a failure. Sleeping pills can sometimes be a lifesaver and that's why they shouldn't be dismissed systematically, especially for temporary use. Certain illnesses or chronic pain can make sleeping pills an absolute necessity. Long-term use of sleeping pills might be problematic, though, especially if taking hypnotic drugs makes you drowsy or makes you feel you are not yourself anymore.

Sleeping pills can sometimes affect the quality of sleep and reduce sleep phases that allow for recovery and regeneration. Someone using sleeping pills might get more hours of sleep each night but less deep sleep because most sleeping pills tend to suppress deep sleep and REM sleep, and promote lighter sleep instead.[13] Because of the many recorded side effects of sleeping pills, the Mayo Clinic recommends that "sleeping pills may help when stress, travel or other disruptions keep you awake. For long-term insomnia, behavior changes learned in behavioral therapy is usually the best treatment."[14]

Additionally, certain sleeping pills are addictive. This means that we will need more and more pills after a while to get the same effect on our insomnia. This is why, ideally, sleeping medicines such as tranquilizers and soporific drugs should only be used temporarily to take care of an acute insomnia episode.

The purpose of this book is to walk you through a non-medicated approach to improving your sleep, so I won't go into detail about the risks and benefits of sleeping pills. Instead, I encourage you to talk to your healthcare provider for more. Ten million French people used sleeping pills in 2018, and an average of 4% of American adults between 2010 and 2015.[15] If, at one point in your life, you have to do it too, you are not alone.

If you have been taking over-the-counter sleep aids or prescription drugs for a while and are considering weaning yourself off them, it is imperative to do so progressively to avoid "rebound insomnia," which is when your sleep becomes even worse than it was before you started taking sleeping pills.[16] It is also critical that you chose a period of your life when things are going well for you: work is not too stressful, your relationships are good, you are not under a lot of pressure, and you feel positive and happy. Trying to quit sleeping pills during a divorce or when you are facing financial hardship is setting yourself up for failure. Just like trying to quit cigarettes or alcohol, it will take time, and it is a journey. Make sure you establish goals and find a profound reason why you are doing it. Working with an expert will help greatly, whether it is a doctor, an addiction coach, a nurse, a therapist, or someone who can help you using cognitive behavioral therapy. You might also want to find support among your loved ones.

Progressing slowly under medical supervision is a safe bet. Talk to your health care provider about taking a little bit less medicine every month rather than decreasing the quantity drastically from one day to another or even from one week to another. Be ready to sleep poorly for several days every time you reduce your meds until your body adjusts to the new situation.[17] Most importantly, treat yourself with all the love and compassion that you would grant someone else. Letting go of sleeping pills is not an easy endeavor, and if you decide to do it, just be proud of yourself for making an effort and getting started on the journey. It will most likely take several attempts and quite a long time to get there. Be patient.

Even if you work with a healthcare professional and resort to external sleeping aids temporarily, understanding how sleep works and what your own sleep needs and obstacles are can only empower you and help you get better results. No matter what your path looks like, I encourage you to go through all the steps of the winning sleep improvement process presented in this book rather than shift the responsibility onto your doctor and put all your hopes into the treatment they might suggest.

Notes

CONCLUSION

I had to hit rock bottom before doing something about my sleep. Illness was the trigger for me to change my ways, and being sick gave me permission to make sleep a priority when everything around and inside me pulled in the other direction. Sleeping didn't come easily to me, and when you are bad at something, you naturally want to stop doing it. Once I understood that quitting was not an option, I had to learn how to become better at it, and I did.

After I'd internalized the fact that I couldn't cut corners, it took me years to assemble the tools and do the work required to improve my sleep. I have made tremendous progress and now sleep well most nights. I went from getting five hours of sleep every night to getting almost eight. Yet, the battle is not over. First, because I need a little more than eight hours to feel rested. Second, because I am still a light sleeper on high alert all the time and need to stay intentional and focused if I want to maintain an environment and lifestyle that promote good sleep. Lastly, and most importantly, because despite everything I know and everything I've told you in this book, my mindset lags. Deep inside, I still have a nagging temptation to skip a few hours of rest here and there to do something more exciting than pass out for eight hours straight. Even as I write this book, I have to resist the urge to squeeze a few more pages into my day and push my sleep to the bottom of my to-do list again. Sleeping well is what I need to do to be who I am. I know this, and I accept it now. This is a significant accomplishment, but it is also a fragile one that needs to be protected on a daily basis.

If you have read this far, I am confident that you recognize the importance of sleep in your life, especially in your health and wellness journey. Without proper rest, weight management, blood sugar control, and an optimal level of performance will most likely remain wishful thinking. I hope that you will now give yourself permission to sleep, even though society tells you otherwise.

Sleep doesn't happen independently from the rest of our lives. So, if you genuinely want to make changes, I also hope that you are now ready to look beyond your bed and the time you spend in it. Among other things, you will have to question your food intake, your values and priorities, your relationships, your financial situation, and more.

By providing you with a step-by-step process and many tools applicable to your everyday life, my goal was to give you the strength and resources to fix your sleep without wasting years, as I did. If I had known years ago that I had the power to sleep well and didn't have to stick to the habits and clichés I grew up with, I would not have suffered from sleep deprivation for decades.

There is no magic pill, no easy recipe. If it were the case, the magic pill would be out there, and we would all take it. As we have seen, different people have different chronotypes, different needs, different circumstances, and a different tolerance threshold for stress or life's mishaps. That's why every single person has to find their very own solution or, I should say, their very own mix of solutions.

Even if this book gives you everything you need to improve your sleep, it will still take time, and it won't be without effort. If you have struggled with your sleep for many years, making changes will require honest soul-searching, mindfulness, and a lot of experimenting. Let me tell you, though: good quality sleep is definitely worth the journey. Not only will it help you reach your health, wellness, and performance goals, but good sleep will also make your whole life better and happier. When we sleep well, we are more tolerant and less cranky and can be present and available for the people in our lives. Our families, friends, and colleagues need us to show up with enough energy to care about our relationships. When we are fully rested, we have the energy to be compassionate and empathetic, something our world desperately needs.

As you move along the winning sleep improvement process presented in this book, it is essential to take your time and give yourself grace while you are making progress. It is already cause for celebration that you are committed enough to have read this book and hopefully completed many of the accompanying worksheets. You have done a big chunk of the work. It is a slow process, and in the same way that you can't reverse prediabetes in two weeks, lose 50 pounds in one month, or prepare for a marathon in 10 days, you cannot expect to fix your sleep overnight. But over time, the benefits add up and you will see the cumulative results from each small step fairly quickly.

Neither acting as a powerless victim nor beating yourself up will help you move forward. It is now time to roll up your sleeves and reach out for help if needed. If you haven't done so yet, download the workbook that will help you do the work and keep all your good work in one place. Start changing your own life one step at a time, acknowledging your progress and focusing on what you achieve rather than what's left to do.

While this book is still fresh in your mind, I encourage you to list your key takeaways and the three most important changes you will make to reach your goals. This is the last worksheet! You can fill it out in your printable workbook, of course, but you can also do it directly online at allonZcoaching. com/sleepitoff and share your answers with me. I would love to hear what you have learned from this book and what you will do with this new awareness. It would also be an opportunity for you to let me know what other tools I could provide to make your success faster and easier.

Now, for all of us trying to improve our sleep, things would be much easier if we were not swimming against the current. Bringing sleep back front and center in our society will take time, but you can help me spread the word! If this book helped you in any way, please consider leaving an honest review on your favorite store's website. Your testimonial could help other readers find the right book for their needs. Thank you for reading and good luck with your sleep. I am going to bed now. Good night!

GET YOUR WORKBOOK AND SPECIAL BONUS!

To download your companion printable Workbook at allonZcoaching.com/sleepitoff, use the exclusive reader's password SLEEP_IT_OFF.

Chances are you have also grabbed what could be an absolute life-saver: the "100 Common Sleep-Killers" checklist. No password needed for that free bonus!

But that's not all...

I have a special bonus for you!

The fact that you are still reading these lines tells me that you are really dedicated to improving your sleep, your health, and your life. For extra support, I have created a delicious **Sample Meal Plan for Better Sleep**, together with a shopping list and recipe booklet.

Grab it now at allonZcoaching.com/sleepitoff and start enjoying delicious meals right away. Bon appétit!

REFERENCES

Chapter 1

1 Mesarwi, Omar, Jan Polak, Jonathan Jun, and Vsevolod Y Polotsky. "Sleep Disorders and the Development of Insulin Resistance and Obesity." Endocrinology and metabolism clinics of North America. U.S. National Library of Medicine, September 2013. https://www.ncbi.nlm.nih.gov/pmc/articles/PMC3767932/.

2 Calhoun, David A, and Susan M Harding. "Sleep and Hypertension." Chest. American College of Chest Physicians, August 2010. https://www.ncbi.nlm.nih.gov/pmc/articles/PMC2913764/.

3 Hirshkowitz M;Whiton K;Albert SM;Alessi C;Bruni O;DonCarlos L;Hazen N;Herman J;Katz ES;Kheirandish-Gozal L;Neubauer DN;O'Donnell AE;Ohayon M;Peever J;Rawding R;Sachdeva RC;Setters B;Vitiello MV;Ware JC;Adams Hillard PJ; "National Sleep Foundation's Sleep Time Duration Recommendations: Methodology and Results Summary." Sleep health. U.S. National Library of Medicine. Accessed August 31, 2020. https://pubmed.ncbi.nlm.nih.gov/29073412/.

4 Tozer, James. "Which Countries Get the Most Sleep?" April 9, 2018. https://www.1843magazine.com/data-graphic/what-the-numbers-say/which-countries-get-the-most-sleep.

5 "Sleep Deprivation and Obesity." The Nutrition Source, July 6, 2015. https://www.hsph.harvard.edu/nutritionsource/sleep/.

6 Beccuti, Guglielmo, and Silvana Pannain. "Sleep and Obesity." Current opinion in clinical nutrition and metabolic care. U.S. National Library of Medicine, July 2011. https://www.ncbi.nlm.nih.gov/pmc/articles/PMC3632337/.

7 Nedetcheva, Arlet V, Jennifer M Kilkus, Jacqueline Imperial, Kristen Kasza, Dale A Schoeller, Plamen D Penev. "Sleep Curtailment Is Accompanied by Increased Intake of Calories from Snacks." OUP Academic. Oxford University Press, December 3, 2008. https://academic.oup.com/ajcn/article/89/1/126/4598230.

8 "Lack of Sleep Disrupts Brain's Emotional Controls." National Institutes of Health. U.S. Department of Health and Human Services, October 5, 2015. https://www.nih.gov/news-events/nih-research-matters/lack-sleep-disrupts-brains-emotional-controls.

9 "What's Behind the Link Between Sleep Deprivation and Type 2 Diabetes." National Sleep Foundation, April 10, 2017. https://www.sleepfoundation.org/articles/link-between-lack-sleep-and-type-2-diabetes.

10 "Losing Sleep Makes It Harder to Lose Fat." American Council on Science and Health, March 27, 2018. https://www.acsh.org/news/2018/03/27/losing-sleep-makes-it-harder-lose-fat-12761.

REFERENCES

11 Vijayakumar, Archana, Ruslan Novosyadlyy, Yingjie Wu, Shoshana Yakar, and Derek LeRoith. "Biological Effects of Growth Hormone on Carbohydrate and Lipid Metabolism." Growth hormone & IGF research: official journal of the Growth Hormone Research Society and the International IGF Research Society. U.S. National Library of Medicine, February 2010. https://www.ncbi.nlm.nih.gov/pmc/articles/PMC2815161/.

12 VanHelder, T, and M W Radomski. "Sleep Deprivation and the Effect on Exercise Performance." Sports medicine (Auckland, N.Z.). U.S. National Library of Medicine, April 1989. https://www.ncbi.nlm.nih.gov/pubmed/2657963.

13 Touma, Carol, and Silvana Pannain. "Does Lack of Sleep Cause Diabetes?" Cleveland Clinic Journal of Medicine. U.S. National Library of Medicine, August 2011. https://www.ncbi.nlm.nih.gov/pubmed/21807927.

14 Easton, John. "New Study Helps Explain Links between Sleep Loss and Diabetes." Science Life, March 9, 2015. https://sciencelife.uchospitals.edu/2015/02/19/new-study-helps-explain-links-between-sleep-loss-and-diabetes/.

15 "The Link Between Lack of Sleep and Type 2 Diabetes." National Sleep Foundation, April 10, 2017. https://www.sleepfoundation.org/articles/link-between-lack-sleep-and-type-2-diabetes

16 Shan, Zhilei, Hongfei Ma, Manling Xie, Peipei Yan, Yanjun Guo, Wei Bao, Ying Rong, Chandra L. Jackson, Frank B. Hu, and Liegang Liu. "Sleep Duration and Risk of Type 2 Diabetes: A Meta-Analysis of Prospective Studies." Diabetes Care. American Diabetes Association, March 1, 2015. https://care.diabetesjournals.org/content/38/3/529.

17 HHS Office, and Council on Sports. "Physical Activity Guidelines for Americans." HHS.gov. US Department of Health and Human Services, February 1, 2019. https://www.hhs.gov/fitness/be-active/physical-activity-guidelines-for-americans/index.html.

18 Lee, Katherine, and Jennifer Warner. "Why Don't Americans Get Enough Sleep?–Everyday Health." EverydayHealth.com. 2014 https://www.everydayhealth.com/news/why-dont-americans-get-enough-sleep/.

19 "Sleep For Success." Sleep For Success. 2020. https://jamesmaas.com/.

20 Van Cauter, E, and L Plat. "Physiology of Growth Hormone Secretion during Sleep." The Journal of Pediatrics. U.S. National Library of Medicine, May 1996. https://www.ncbi.nlm.nih.gov/pubmed/8627466.

21 Godfrey, Richard J, Zahra Madgwick, and Gregory P Whyte. "The Exercise-Induced Growth Hormone Response in Athletes." Sports Medicine (Auckland, N.Z.). U.S. National Library of Medicine, 2003. https://www.ncbi.nlm.nih.gov/pubmed/12797841.

22 Saugy, M, N Robinson, C Saudan, N Baume, L Avois, and P Mangin. "Human Growth Hormone Doping in Sport." British Journal of Sports Medicine. BMJ Group, July 2006. https://www.ncbi.nlm.nih.gov/pmc/articles/PMC2657499/.

23 "Human Growth Hormone (HGH) Testing." World Anti-Doping Agency, July 29, 2015. https://www.wada-ama.org/en/questions-answers/human-growth-hormone-hgh-testing.

24 Welle, S, C Thornton, M Statt, and B McHenry. "Growth Hormone Increases Muscle Mass and Strength but Does Not Rejuvenate Myofibrillar Protein Synthesis in Healthy Subjects over 60 Years Old." The Journal of Clinical Endocrinology and Metabolism. U.S. National Library of Medicine, September 1996. https://www.ncbi.nlm.nih.gov/pubmed/8784075.

25 How Do Muscles Grow? 2004. https://www.unm.edu/~lkravitz/Article folder/musclesgrowLK.html.

26 Growth Hormone (Somatotropin) 2018. http://www.vivo.colostate.edu/hbooks/pathphys/endocrine/hypopit/gh.html.

27 "Can Triglycerides Affect My Heart Health?" Mayo Clinic. Mayo Foundation for Medical Education and Research, September 13, 2018. https://www.mayoclinic.org/diseases-conditions/high-blood-cholesterol/in-depth/triglycerides/art-20048186.

28 Dimitrov, Stoyan, Tanja Lange, Cécile Gouttefangeas, Anja T R Jensen, et al. "Gαs-Coupled Receptor Signaling and Sleep Regulate Integrin Activation of Human Antigen-Specific T Cells." Journal of Experimental Medicine. The Rockefeller University Press, March 4, 2019. http://jem.rupress.org/content/216/3/517.

29 "Sleep Debt Hikes Risk of Stroke Symptoms despite Healthy BMI–News." UAB News, June 11, 2012. https://www.uab.edu/news/health/item/2483-sleep-debt-hikes-risk-of-stroke-symptoms-despite-healthy-bmi.

30 Cappuccio, Francesco P, and Michelle A Miller. "Sleep and Cardio-Metabolic Disease." Current cardiology reports. Springer US, September 19, 2017. https://www.ncbi.nlm.nih.gov/pmc/articles/PMC5605599/.

31 "Sleep Loss Encourages Spread of Toxic Alzheimer's Protein." National Institute on Aging. U.S. Department of Health and Human Services, February 2019. https://www.nia.nih.gov/news/sleep-loss-encourages-spread-toxic-alzheimers-protein.

32 "Brain May Flush out Toxins during Sleep." September 17, 2015. https://www.nih.gov/news-events/news-releases/brain-may-flush-out-toxins-during-sleep.

33 "Lack of Sleep May Be Linked to Risk Factor for Alzheimer's Disease." National Institutes of Health. U.S. Department of Health and Human Services, April 13, 2018. https://www.nih.gov/news-events/lack-sleep-may-be-linked-risk-factor-alzheimers-disease.

34 Wichniak, Adam, Aleksandra Wierzbicka, Małgorzata Walęcka, and Wojciech Jernajczyk. "Effects of Antidepressants on Sleep," August 9, 2017. https://www.ncbi.nlm.nih.gov/pmc/articles/PMC5548844/.

35 "A Quoi Sert Le Sommeil ?" France Inter, July 2, 2019. https://www.franceinter.fr/emissions/grand-bien-vous-fasse/grand-bien-vous-fasse-02-juillet-2019.

Chapter 2

1 Zoldan, Rachel Jacoby. "This Is What Actually Happens To Your Body When You Don't Get Enough Sleep." SELF. March 10, 2016. https://www.self.com/story/this-is-what-actually-happens-to-your-body-when-you-dont-get-enough-sleep.

2 "Sleep and Health." World Health Organization. World Health Organization, World Federation of Sleep Research Societies, 1998. https://apps.who.int/iris/bitstream/handle/10665/64100/WHO_MSA_MND_98.3.pdf?sequence=1&isAllowed=y.

3 Solly, Meilan. "Nearly One-Third of Americans Sleep Fewer Than Six Hours Per Night." Smithsonian.com. Smithsonian Institution, December 26, 2018. https://www.smithsonianmag.com/smart-news/almost-one-third-americans-sleep-fewer-six-hours-night-180971116/.

4 Sheehan, Connor M, Stephen E Frochen, and Jennifer A Ailshire. "Are U.S. Adults Reporting Less Sleep?: Findings from Sleep Duration Trends in the National Health Interview Survey, 2004–2017." OUP Academic. Oxford University Press, November 17, 2018. https://academic.oup.com/sleep/advance-article-abstract/doi/10.1093/sleep/zsy221/5185637?redirectedFrom=fulltext.

5 Atlantico, Rédaction. "Debout à 7h ? 67% Des Français Se Lèvent plus Tard Que Vous (Mais Seulement 43 % Des Japonais) : L'infographie Qui Vous Dit Qui Se Lève Et Se Couche Quand." Atlantico.fr, August 26, 2014. https://www.atlantico.fr/decryptage/1716554/debout-a-7h—67-des-francais-se-levent-plus-tard-que-vous-mais-seulement-43-des-japonais—l-infographie-qui-vous-dit-qui-se-leve-et-se-couche-quand.

6 Lazovick, Meg. "WAKE ME UP: What Time Do Americans Start Their Day?" Edison Research. Meg Lazovick http://www.edisonresearch.com/wp-content/uploads/2014/06/edison-logo-300x137.jpg, June 29, 2016. https://www.edisonresearch.com/wake-me-up-series-2/.

7 Kluger, Jeffrey. "Sleep: See How Different Countries Sleep."Time. Time, May 6, 2016. https://time.com/4318156/sleep-countries-style/.

8 "About the ESS." Epworth Sleepiness Scale, 2020. http://epworthsleepinessscale.com/about-the-ess/.

9 Smith, Yolanda. "Spoon Test for Sleep Deprivation." News, August 23, 2018. https://www.news-medical.net/health/Spoon-Test-for-Sleep-Deprivation.aspx.

Chapter 3

1 Gul, Somia. "Rapid Eye Movement and Sleep Twitches Can Enhance Brain Activity." Research and Reviews in Pharmacy and Pharmaceutical Sciences, December 25, 2015. http://www.rroij.com/open-access/rapid-eye-movement-and-sleep-twitches-can-enhance-brain-activity-.php?aid=67103.

2 "Sleep 101 Basics: REM, NREM, Sleep Stages, & More." Cleveland Clinic, 2012. https://my.clevelandclinic.org/health/articles/12148-sleep-basics.

3 Length of Circadian Cycle in Humans–Circadian Sleep Disorders Network, 2020. https://www.circadiansleepdisorders.org/info/cycle_length.php.

4 Cromie, William J. "Human Biological Clock Set Back an Hour." Harvard Gazette. Harvard Gazette, September 20, 2016. https://news.harvard.edu/gazette/story/1999/07/human-biological-clock-set-back-an-hour/.

5 Dubuc, Bruno. "Chronobiology."THE BRAIN FROM TOP TO BOTTOM, 2002. https://thebrain.mcgill.ca/flash/a/a_11/a_11_p/a_11_p_hor/a_11_p_hor.html.

6 Méan, Dominique. *Devenez L'acteur De Votre Sommeil*. Bruxelles: Genèse Edition, 2018.

7 Lack, Leon, Michelle Bailey, Nicole Lovato, and Helen Wright. "Chronotype Differences in Circadian Rhythms of Temperature, Melatonin, and Sleepiness as Measured in a Modified Constant Routine Protocol." Nature and Science of Sleep. Dove Medical Press, November 4, 2009. https://www.ncbi.nlm.nih.gov/pmc/articles/PMC3630920/.

8 Biggs, Sarah. "Are You a Night Owl or an Early Bird?" Sleep Health Foundation. International Journal of Chronobiology, Monash University, 2015. http://www.sleephealthfoundation.org.au/pdfs/World Sleep Day/Activity–Morning-Eveningness Questionnaire.pdf

9 Fischer, Dorothee, David A Lombardi, Helen Marucci-Wellman, and Till Roenneberg. "Chronotypes in the US–Influence of Age and Sex." PloS one. Public Library of Science, June 21, 2017. https://www.ncbi.nlm.nih.gov/pmc/articles/PMC5479630/.

10 Beaulieu, Dr. Philippe, and Dr. Olivier Pallanca. *Dormir sans Médoc Et Ni Tisanes. Les Nouvelles Solutions De La Médecine Du Sommeil*. Marabout, 2018.

11 Karasek, M. "Melatonin, Human Aging, and Age-Related Diseases." Experimental Gerontology. U.S. National Library of Medicine, 2004. https://www.ncbi.nlm.nih.gov/pubmed/15582288.

12 "A Quoi Sert Le Sommeil ?" France Inter, July 2, 2019. https://www.franceinter.fr/emissions/grand-bien-vous-fasse/grand-bien-vous-fasse-02-juillet-2019.

13 Devlin, Hannah. "Restless Development: Bad Sleep May Be Evolutionary Survival Tool, Study Finds."The Guardian. Guardian News and Media, July 12, 2017. https://www.theguardian.com/science/2017/jul/12/bad-sleep-evolution-survival.

14 Boubekri, Mohamed, Ivy N. Cheung, Chia-Hui Wang, Kathryn J. Reid, and Phyllis C. Zee,. "Impact of Windows and Daylight Exposure on Overall Health and Sleep Quality of Office Workers: A Case-Control Pilot Study." Journal of Clinical Sleep Medicine, June 15, 2014. https://jcsm.aasm.org/doi/10.5664/jcsm.3780.\

15 "Boosting Your Serotonin Activity." Psychology Today. Sussex Publishers, November 17, 2011. https://www.psychologytoday.com/us/blog/prefrontal-nudity/201111/boosting-your-serotonin-activity.

16 "Serotonin: Facts, Uses, SSRIs, and Sources." Medical News Today. MediLexicon International, 2020. https://www.medicalnewstoday.com/articles/232248.

17 Sylwester, Robert. "The Neurobiology of Self-Esteem and Aggression." Educational Leadership, November 30, 1996. https://eric.ed.gov/?id=EJ539095.

18 Jillian Avey, Certified Executive and Performance Coach, Jillian Avey Coaching, https://aveycoach.com/

19 Uvnas-Moberg, Kerstin, and Maria Petersson. "Oxytocin, a Mediator of Anti-Stress, Well-Being, Social Interaction, Growth and Healing." Zeitschrift fur Psychosomatische Medizin und Psychotherapie. U.S. National Library of Medicine, 2005. https://www.ncbi.nlm.nih.gov/pubmed/15834840.

20 Salamon, Maureen. "11 Interesting Effects of Oxytocin." LiveScience. Purch, May 30, 2013. https://www.livescience.com/35219-11-effects-of-oxytocin.html.

Chapter 4

1 Dubuc, Bruno. "MOLECULES THAT BUILD UP AND MAKE YOU SLEEP." THE BRAIN FROM TOP TO BOTTOM, 2002. https://thebrain.mcgill.ca/flash/i/i_11/i_11_m/i_11_m_cyc/i_11_m_cyc.html.

2 "Does Exercise Help or Hurt Sleep?" Sleep.org. National Sleep Foundation, 2020. https://www.sleep.org/articles/does-exercise-help-or-hurt-sleep/

3 Dworak, M, P Diel, S Voss, W Hollmann, and H K Strüder. "Intense Exercise Increases Adenosine Concentrations in Rat Brain: Implications for a Homeostatic Sleep Drive." Neuroscience. U.S. National Library of Medicine, December 19, 2007. https://www.ncbi.nlm.nih.gov/pubmed/18031936.

4 Ekirch, A Roger. "Segmented Sleep in Preindustrial Societies," March 1, 2016. https://www.ncbi.nlm.nih.gov/pmc/articles/PMC4763365/.

5 Max, M and M. Menaker. "Regulation of Melatonin Production by Light, Darkness, and Temperature in the Trout Pineal." Journal of Comparative Physiology A: Sensory, neural, and behavioral physiology. U.S. National Library of Medicine, April 1992. https://www.ncbi.nlm.nih.gov/pubmed/1625220.

6 Landsberg, Lewis, James B Young, William R Leonard, Robert A Linsenmeier, and Fred W Turek. "Do the Obese Have Lower Body Temperatures? A New Look at a Forgotten Variable in Energy Balance." Transactions of the American Clinical and Climatological Association. American Clinical and Climatological Association, 2009. https://www.ncbi.nlm.nih.gov/pmc/articles/PMC2744512/.

7 Raymann, Roy J E M, Dick F Swaab, and Eus J W Van Someren. "Skin Deep: Enhanced Sleep Depth by Cutaneous Temperature Manipulation." Brain : a Journal of Neurology. U.S. National Library of Medicine, February 2008. https://www.ncbi.nlm.nih.gov/pubmed/18192289.

8 Obradovich, Nick, Robyn Migliorini, Sara C. Mednick, and James H. Fowler. "Nighttime Temperature and Human Sleep Loss in a Changing Climate." Science Advances. American Association for the Advancement of Science, May 1, 2017. https://advances.sciencemag.org/content/3/5/e1601555.

9 Breus, Michael. "Understanding GABA." Your Guide to Better Sleep, January 4, 2019. https://thesleepdoctor.com/2018/06/19/understanding-gaba/.

10 Gottesmann, Claude. "GABA Mechanisms and Sleep." Neuroscience. U.S. National Library of Medicine, 2002. https://www.ncbi.nlm.nih.gov/pubmed/11983310.

Chapter 5

1 "Insomnia." Mayo Clinic. Mayo Foundation for Medical Education and Research, October 15, 2016. https://www.mayoclinic.org/diseases-conditions/insomnia/symptoms-causes/syc-20355167.

2 Roth, Thomas. "Insomnia: Definition, Prevalence, Etiology, and Consequences." Journal of Clinical Sleep Medicine : JCSM : official publication of the American Academy of Sleep Medicine. American Academy of Sleep Medicine, August 15, 2007. https://www.ncbi.nlm.nih.gov/pmc/articles/PMC1978319/.

3 "Insomnia." womenshealth.gov, November 21, 2018. https://www.womenshealth.gov/a-z-topics/insomnia.

4 "The Complex Relationship Between Sleep, Depression & Anxiety." National Sleep Foundation, 2020. https://www.sleepfoundation.org/excessive-sleepiness/health-impact/complex-relationship-between-sleep-depression-anxiety.

5 "Sleep and Mental Health." Harvard Health. Harvard Health Publishing, July 2009. https://www.health.harvard.edu/newsletter_article/Sleep-and-mental-health.

6 "Too Early to Get up, Too Late to Get Back to Sleep." Harvard Health. Harvard Health Publishing, June 2010. https://www.health.harvard.edu/staying-healthy/too-early-to-get-up-too-late-to-get-back-to-sleep.

7 Wichniak, Adam, Aleksandra Wierzbicka, Małgorzata Wal□cka, and Wojciech Jernajczyk. "Effects of Antidepressants on Sleep," August 9, 2017. https://www.ncbi.nlm.nih.gov/pmc/articles/PMC5548844/.

8 Chronic Conditions Team. "How to Beat Insomnia When You Have Chronic Pain." Health Essentials from Cleveland Clinic. Health Essentials from Cleveland Clinic, May 8, 2020. https://health.clevelandclinic.org/managing-insomnia-for-those-with-chronic-pain/.

9 Moore, Jason T, and Max B Kelz. "Opiates, Sleep, and Pain: the Adenosinergic Link." Anesthesiology. U.S. National Library of Medicine, December 2009. https://www.ncbi.nlm.nih.gov/pmc/articles/PMC2784658/.

10 "Antidepressants: Get Tips to Cope with Side Effects." Mayo Clinic. Mayo Foundation for Medical Education and Research, September 12, 2019. https://www.mayoclinic.org/diseases-conditions/depression/in-depth/antidepressants/art-20049305.

11 Moustakas, Dimitrios, Michael Mezzio, Branden R Rodriguez, Mic Andre Constable, Margaret E Mulligan, and Evelyn B Voura. "Guarana Provides Additional Stimulation over Caffeine Alone in the Planarian Model." PloS One. Public Library of Science, April 16, 2015. https://www.ncbi.nlm.nih.gov/pmc/articles/PMC4399916/).

12 "Caffeine and Sleep–How Long Coffee Stays in the Body." Sleep Advisor, May 11, 2020. https://www.sleepadvisor.org/caffeine-and-sleep/.

13 Cappelletti, Simone, Daria Piacentino, Gabriele Sani, and Mariarosaria Aromatario. "Caffeine: Cognitive and Physical Performance Enhancer or Psychoactive Drug?" Current neuropharmacology. Bentham Science Publishers, January 2015. https://www.ncbi.nlm.nih.gov/pmc/articles/PMC4462044/.

14 "Caffeine Content for Coffee, Tea, Soda, and More" Mayo Clinic. Mayo Foundation for Medical Education and Research, February 29, 2020. https://www.mayoclinic.org/healthy-lifestyle/nutrition-and-healthy-eating/in-depth/caffeine/art-20049372.

15 Drake, Christopher, Timothy Roehrs, John Shambroom, and Thomas Roth. "Caffeine Effects on Sleep Taken 0, 3, or 6 Hours before Going to Bed." Journal of Clinical Sleep Medicine, November 15, 2013. http://jcsm.aasm.org/viewabstract.aspx?pid=29198.

16 Kruszelnicki, Karl S. "Why Does Drinking Alcohol Cause Dehydration?" ABC, February 28, 2012. https://www.abc.net.au/science/articles/2012/02/28/3441707.htm.

17 Sagawa, Yohei, Hideaki Kondo, Namiko Matsubuchi, Takaubu Takemura, Hironobu Kanayama, Yoshihiko Kaneko, Takashi Kanbayashi, Yasuo Hishikawa, and Tetsuo Shimizu. "Alcohol Has a Dose-Related Effect on Parasympathetic Nerve Activity During Sleep." Wiley Online Library. John Wiley & Sons, Ltd, August 16, 2011. https://onlinelibrary.wiley.com/doi/abs/10.1111/j.1530-0277.2011.01558.x.

18 Conroy, Deirdre A, Megan E Kurth, David R Strong, Kirk J Brower, and Michael D Stein. "Marijuana Use Patterns and Sleep among Community-Based Young Adults." Journal of Addictive Diseases. U.S. National Library of Medicine, 2016. https://www.ncbi.nlm.nih.gov/pmc/articles/PMC4911998/.

19 Gregoire, Carolyn. "A Surprising New Link Between Stress And Weight." HuffPost. HuffPost, June 20, 2013. https://www.huffpost.com/entry/stress-weight-gain_n_3459755.

20 EndoMedia. "Being Overweight Linked to Excess Stress Hormones after Eating." EurekAlert!, June 15, 2013. https://www.eurekalert.org/pub_releases/2013-06/tes-bol061513.php.

21 Franklin, Karl A, and Eva Lindberg. "Obstructive Sleep Apnea Is a Common Disorder in the Population–a Review on the Epidemiology of Sleep Apnea." Journal of Thoracic Disease. AME Publishing Company, August 2015. https://www.ncbi.nlm.nih.gov/pmc/articles/PMC4561280/.

22 Epstein, Lawrence J, David Kristo, Patrick J Strollo, Norman Friedman, Atul Malhotra, Susheel P Patil, Kannan Ramar, et al. "Clinical Guideline for the Evaluation, Management and Long-Term Care of Obstructive Sleep Apnea in Adults." Journal of Clinical Sleep Medicine : JCSM : official publication of the American Academy of Sleep Medicine. American Academy of Sleep Medicine, June 15, 2009. https://www.ncbi.nlm.nih.gov/pmc/articles/PMC2699173/.

23 "Restless Legs Syndrome Fact Sheet." National Institute of Neurological Disorders and Stroke. U.S. Department of Health and Human Services, May 2017. https://www.ninds.nih.gov/Disorders/Patient-Caregiver-Education/Fact-Sheets/Restless-Legs-Syndrome-Fact-Sheet.

Chapter 6

1 "Microbes Help Produce Serotonin in Gut." California Institute of Technology, April 9, 2015. https://www.caltech.edu/about/news/microbes-help-produce-serotonin-gut-46495.

2 Smith, Robert P, Cole Easson, Sarah M Lyle, Ritishka Kapoor, Chase P Donnelly, Eileen J Davidson, Esha Parikh, Jose V Lopez, and Jaime L Tartar. "Gut Microbiome Diversity Is Associated with Sleep Physiology in Humans." PloS One. Public Library of Science, October 7, 2019. https://www.ncbi.nlm.nih.gov/pmc/articles/PMC6779243/.

3 "What Is Tryptophan?" Sleep.org, 2020. https://www.sleep.org/articles/what-is-tryptophan/.

4 HHS Office, and Council on Sports. "Facts & Statistics." HHS.gov. US Department of Health and Human Services, January 26, 2017. https://www.hhs.gov/fitness/resource-center/facts-and-statistics/index.html.

5 "Physical Activity." World Health Organization. World Health Organization, February 23, 2018. https://www.who.int/news-room/fact-sheets/detail/physical-activity.

6 Christine Suter, Professional Life Coach, MA, CPC, www.affirmationinaction.com

Chapter 7

1 Leger, Damien. "Les Thérapies Contre Les Troubles Du Sommeil Deviennent Efficaces." Le Figaro Santé, 2019.

2 "Nicotine." Psychology Today. Sussex Publishers, March 26, 2019. https://www.psychologytoday.com/us/conditions/nicotine.

3 Ashton, H, J E Milliman, R Telford, and J W Thompson. "Stimulant and Depressant Effects of Cigarette Smoking on Brain Activity in Man." British Journal of Pharmacology. U.S. National Library of Medicine, August 1973. https://www.ncbi.nlm.nih.gov/pmc/articles/PMC1776143/.

4 Young, Simon N. "How to Increase Serotonin in the Human Brain without Drugs." Journal of Psychiatry & Neuroscience : JPN. Canadian Medical Association, November 2007. https://www.ncbi.nlm.nih.gov/pmc/articles/PMC2077351/.

5 Dolezal, Brett A, Eric V Neufeld, David M Boland, Jennifer L Martin, and Christopher B Cooper. "Interrelationship between Sleep and Exercise: A Systematic Review." Advances in Preventive Medicine. Hindawi, 2017. https://www.ncbi.nlm.nih.gov/pmc/articles/PMC5385214/.

6 Laborde, Sylvain, Thomas Hosang, Emma Mosley, and Fabrice Dosseville. "Influence of a 30-Day Slow-Paced Breathing Intervention Compared to Social Media Use on Subjective Sleep Quality and Cardiac Vagal Activity." Journal of Clinical Medicine. MDPI, February 6, 2019. https://www.ncbi.nlm.nih.gov/pmc/articles/PMC6406675/.

7 Christopher Hill, Doctor of Chiropractic, https://www.newbalancechiropractic.com/

8 "Cannabidiol" Expert Committee on Drug Dependence. World Health Organization, November 2017. https://www.who.int/medicines/access/controlled-substances/5.2_CBD.pdf

9 ASA Authors & Reviewers Sleep Physician, and American Sleep Association Reviewers. "CBD: For Sleep and Insomnia." American Sleep Association, 2020. https://www.sleepassociation.org/sleep-treatments/cbd/.

10 Grinspoon, Peter. "Cannabidiol (CBD)—What We Know and What We Don't." Harvard Health Blog, April 22, 2020. https://www.health.harvard.edu/blog/cannabidiol-cbd-what-we-know-and-what-we-dont-2018082414476.

11 "Quick Coherence Technique for Adults." HeartMath Institute, 2020. https://www.heartmath.org/resources/heartmath-tools/quick-coherence-technique-for-adults/.

12 Harvard Health Publishing. "Therapy Beats Drugs for Chronic Insomnia." Harvard Health, June 2016. https://www.health.harvard.edu/diseases-and-conditions/therapy-beats-drugs-for-chronic-insomnia.

13 Mary Torres, Licensed Mental Health Counselor and Nationally Certified Counselor (MA, LMHC, NCC), Founder of Cornerstone OCD and Anxiety in Seattle. www.CornerstoneOCD.com

14 Anthony Gitch, Board Certified Clinical Hypnotherapist affiliated with the International Certification Board of Clinical Hypnotherapists (ICBCH) excelhypnosis.com

15 U.S. Department of Health and Human Services, May 2016. https://www.nccih.nih.gov/health/relaxation-techniques-for-health.

16 Tainya C. Clarke, Ph.D., M.P.H.; Patricia M. Barnes, M.A.; Lindsey I. Black, M.P.H.; Barbara J. Stussman, B.A.; and Richard L. Nahin, Ph.D., M.P.H. "Use of Yoga, Meditation, and Chiropractors Among U.S. Adults Aged 18 and Over." CDC, November 2018. https://www.cdc.gov/nchs/data/databriefs/db325-h.pdf

17 Black, David S. "Mindfulness Meditation in Sleep-Disturbed Adults." JAMA Internal Medicine. American Medical Association, April 1, 2015. https://jamanetwork.com/journals/jamainternalmedicine/fullarticle/2110998.

18 "Brain Waves and Meditation." ScienceDaily. ScienceDaily, March 31, 2010. https://www.sciencedaily.com/releases/2010/03/100319210631.htm.

19 Nancy K Ishii, LAc AEMP, Acupuncture at Grace Unfolding PLLC, www.ishiiacupuncture.com

20 National Certification Commission for Acupuncture and Oriental Medicine. nccaom.org, 2020. https://www.nccaom.org/find-a-practitioner-directory/.

21 Shariati, A., S. Jahani, M. Hooshmand, and N. Khalili. "The Effect of Acupressure on Sleep Quality in Hemodialysis Patients." Complementary Therapies in Medicine. Churchill Livingstone, August 31, 2012. https://www.sciencedirect.com/science/article/abs/pii/S0965229912001161.

22 Lu, Mei-Jou. "Acupressure Improves Sleep Quality of Psychogeriatric… : Nursing Research." LWW, 2013. https://journals.lww.com/nursingresearchonline/Abstract/2013/03000/Acupressure_Improves_Sleep_Quality_of.9.aspx.

23 "Aromatherapy: Do Essential Oils Really Work?" Aromatherapy: Do Essential Oils Really Work? | Johns Hopkins Medicine, 2020. https://www.hopkinsmedicine.org/health/wellness-and-prevention/aromatherapy-do-essential-oils-really-work.

24 "A Systematic Review of the Effect of Inhaled Essential Oils on Sleep." Database of Abstracts of Reviews of Effects (DARE): Quality-assessed Reviews [Internet]. U.S. National Library of Medicine, January 1, 1970. https://www.ncbi.nlm.nih.gov/books/NBK246974/.

25 Koulivand, Peir Hossein, Maryam Khaleghi Ghadiri, and Ali Gorji. "Lavender and the Nervous System." Evidence-based Complementary and Alternative Medicine : eCAM. Hindawi Publishing Corporation, 2013. https://www.ncbi.nlm.nih.gov/pmc/articles/PMC3612440/.

26 Elise Kloter, Massage Therapist (MT), Owner of Lotus Massage https://elisekloter.amtamembers.com/

27 Moraska, Albert, Robin Pollini, Karen Boulanger, Marissa Brooks, and Lesley Teitlebaum. Physiological Adjustments to Stress Measures Following Massage Therapy: A Review of the Literature. NCBI, National Institutes of Health, May 7, 2008. https://www.ncbi.nlm.nih.gov/pmc/articles/PMC2892349/.

28 "National Certification Board for Therapeutic Massage & Bodywork." NCBTMB, June 22, 2020. https://www.ncbtmb.org/.

29 American Massage Therapy Association, AMTA, 2020. https://www.amtamassage.org/

30 Associated Bodywork & Massage Professionals, ABMP, 2020. https://www.abmp.com/.

31 Breus, Michael. "The Sleep Doctor's 5 Relaxation Techniques to Help You De-Stress and Sleep Better." Your Guide to Better Sleep, November 20, 2016. https://thesleepdoctor.com/2016/11/19/sleep-doctors-5-relaxation-techniques-help-de-stress-sleep-better/.

32 "Relaxation Techniques for Health." National Center for Complementary and Integrative Health. U.S. Department of Health and Human Services, May 2016. https://www.nccih.nih.gov/health/relaxation-techniques-for-health.

33 "Relaxation Exercises for Falling Asleep." National Sleep Foundation, April 28, 2020. https://www.sleepfoundation.org/articles/relaxation-exercises-falling-asleep.

34 Jennings, Kerri-Ann. "16 Simple Ways to Relieve Stress and Anxiety." Healthline. Healthline Media, August 28, 2018. https://www.healthline.com/nutrition/16-ways-relieve-stress-anxiety.

35 "Yoga for Sleep." Yoga for Sleep | Johns Hopkins Medicine, 2020. https://www.hopkinsmedicine.org/health/wellness-and-prevention/yoga-for-sleep.

36 Sharpe, Erica. "A Closer Look at Yoga Nidra: Sleep Lab Analyses." National University of Natural Medicine. Helfgott Research Institute. August 29th, 2018 https://www.clinicaltrials.gov/ProvidedDocs/27/NCT03685227/Prot_SAP_000.pdf

37 Tamara Gillest, Certified Yoga Therapist (C-IAYT), Founder and Owner of BendnMove, https://bendnmove.com/

38 Bankar, Mangesh A, Sarika K Chaudhari, and Kiran D Chaudhari. "Impact of Long-Term Yoga Practice on Sleep Quality and Quality of Life in the Elderly." Journal of Ayurveda and Integrative Medicine. Medknow Publications & Media Pvt Ltd, January 2013. https://www.ncbi.nlm.nih.gov/pmc/articles/PMC3667430/.

39 Caldwell, JL. "Non-Traditional Methods for the Treatment of Insomnia: A Mini Review." Austin Journal of Sleep Disorders, 2015. https://austinpublishinggroup.com/sleep-disorders/fulltext/ajsd-v2-id1007.php.

40 "Do You Have Chronic Dehydration?" University Health News, December 16, 2019. https://universityhealthnews.com/daily/nutrition/do-you-have-chronic-dehydration/.

41 "More Than Just a Fad: 4 Ways Weighted Blankets Can Actually Help You." Penn Medicine, February 5, 2019. https://www.pennmedicine.org/updates/blogs/health-and-wellness/2019/february/weighted-blankets.

42 Regen, Isalou. Le Magie Du Sommeil. Vivre Et Dormir Enfin!, 2018.

43 Wurtman, R J, and J J Wurtman. "Brain Serotonin, Carbohydrate-Craving, Obesity and Depression." Obesity Research. U.S. National Library of Medicine, November 1995. https://www.ncbi.nlm.nih.gov/pubmed/8697046.

Chapter 8

1 Lee, Jinju, Youngsin Han, Hyun Hee Cho, and Mee-Ran Kim. "Sleep Disorders and Menopause." Journal of Menopausal Medicine. The Korean Society of Menopause, August 2019. https://www.ncbi.nlm.nih.gov/pmc/articles/PMC6718648/.

2 "How Does Menopause Affect My Sleep?" How Does Menopause Affect My Sleep? | Johns Hopkins Medicine, 2020. https://www.hopkinsmedicine.org/health/wellness-and-prevention/how-does-menopause-affect-my-sleep.

3 "Menopause & Sleep." National Sleep Foundation, April 17, 2009. https://www.sleepfoundation.org/articles/menopause-and-sleep.

4 "Straight Talk About Soy." The Nutrition Source, October 28, 2019. https://www.hsph.harvard.edu/nutritionsource/soy/.

5 Dastjerdi, Marziyeh, Bita Eslami, Maryam Alsadat Sharifi, Ashraf Moini, Leila Bayani, Hoda Mohammad Khani, and Sadaf Alipour. "Effect of Soy Isoflavone on Hot Flushes, Endometrial Thickness, and Breast Clinical as Well as Sonographic Features." Iranian Journal of Public Health. Tehran University of Medical Sciences, March 2018. https://www.ncbi.nlm.nih.gov/pmc/articles/PMC5971175/.

6 "TMHS 225: The Truth about Naps & Sleep Tips for Parents." The Model Health Show, 2020. https://themodelhealthshow.com/the-truth-about-naps/.

7 "Debunking Sleep Myths: Does Napping During the Day Affect Your Sleep at Night?" National Sleep Foundation, July 20, 2018. https://www.sleepfoundation.org/articles/debunking-sleep-myths-does-napping-during-day-affect-your-sleep-night.

8 Malleret, Thierry. "Night-Shift Work Is on the Rise Globally – and It's a New Wellness Problem." Global Wellness Institute, July 5, 2018. https://globalwellnessinstitute.org/global-wellness-institute-blog/2018/06/19/night-shift-work-is-on-the-rise-globally-and-its-a-new-wellness-problem/.

9 "Work Schedules: Shift Work and Long Hours." Centers for Disease Control and Prevention, August 29, 2018. https://www.cdc.gov/niosh/topics/workschedules/default.html.

10 Institute of Medicine (US) Committee on Military Nutrition Research. "Pharmacology of Caffeine." Caffeine for the Sustainment of Mental Task Performance: Formulations for Military Operations. U.S. National Library of Medicine, January 1, 1970. https://www.ncbi.nlm.nih.gov/books/NBK223808/.

Chapter 9

1 Herroeder, Susanne, Marianne E. Schönherr, Stefan G. De Hert, and Markus W. Hollmann. "Magnesium-Essentials for Anesthesiologists." Anesthesiology. The American Society of Anesthesiologists, April 1, 2011. https://anesthesiology.pubs.asahq.org/article.aspx?articleid=1930758.

2 Sartori, S B, N Whittle, A Hetzenauer, and N Singewald. "Magnesium Deficiency Induces Anxiety and HPA Axis Dysregulation: Modulation by Therapeutic Drug Treatment." Neuropharmacology. Pergamon Press, January 2012. https://www.ncbi.nlm.nih.gov/pmc/articles/PMC3198864/.

3 Eby, George A. "Magnesium and Major Depression." Magnesium in the Central Nervous System [Internet]. U.S. National Library of Medicine, January 1, 1970. https://www.ncbi.nlm.nih.gov/books/NBK507265/.

4 "Muscle Cramp." Mayo Clinic. Mayo Foundation for Medical Education and Research, January 3, 2019. https://www.mayoclinic.org/diseases-conditions/muscle-cramp/symptoms-causes/syc-20350820.

5 "Office of Dietary Supplements–Magnesium." NIH Office of Dietary Supplements. U.S. Department of Health and Human Services, March 24, 2020. https://ods.od.nih.gov/factsheets/Magnesium-HealthProfessional/.

6 "22 Low Magnesium Symptoms." University Health News, April 1, 2020. https://universityhealthnews.com/daily/pain/low-magnesium-symptoms-are-these-a-clue-to-the-cause-of-your-health-problem/.

7 Center for Food Safety and Applied Nutrition. "Dietary Supplements." U.S. Food and Drug Administration. FDA. 2020. https://www.fda.gov/food/dietary-supplements.

8 Erland, Lauren A E, and Praveen K Saxena. "Melatonin Natural Health Products and Supplements: Presence of Serotonin and Significant Variability of Melatonin Content." Journal of Clinical Sleep Medicine : JCSM : official publication of the American Academy of Sleep Medicine. American Academy of Sleep Medicine, February 15, 2017. https://www.ncbi.nlm.nih.gov/pubmed/27855744.

9 Gooneratne, Nalaka S. "Complementary and Alternative Medicine for Sleep Disturbances in Older Adults." Clinics in Geriatric Medicine. U.S. National Library of Medicine, February 2008. https://www.ncbi.nlm.nih.gov/pmc/articles/PMC2276624/.

10 Bauer, Brent. "Herbal Treatment for Anxiety: Is It Effective?" Mayo Clinic. Mayo Foundation for Medical Education and Research, March 2, 2018. https://www.mayoclinic.org/diseases-conditions/generalized-anxiety-disorder/expert-answers/herbal-treatment-for-anxiety/faq-20057945.

11 Thomson, Elizabeth A. "Rest Easy: MIT Study Confirms Melatonin's Value as Sleep Aid." MIT News, March 1, 2005. http://news.mit.edu/2005/melatonin.

12 "Herbal Supplements: What to Know before You Buy." Mayo Clinic. Mayo Foundation for Medical Education and Research, November 8, 2017. https://www.mayoclinic.org/healthy-lifestyle/nutrition-and-healthy-eating/in-depth/herbal-supplements/art-20046714.

13 Science-et-vie.com. "Les Somnifères : Tout Ce Qu'il Faut Savoir En 5 Questions." Science, February 12, 2019. https://www.science-et-vie.com/corps-et-sante/les-somniferes-tout-ce-qu-il-faut-savoir-en-5-questions-8428.

14 "Prescription Sleeping Pills: What's Right for You?" Mayo Clinic. Mayo Foundation for Medical Education and Research, January 30, 2018. https://www.mayoclinic.org/diseases-conditions/insomnia/in-depth/sleeping-pills/art-20043959.

15 "Products–Data Briefs–Number 127–August 2013." Centers for Disease Control and Prevention., November 6, 2015. https://www.cdc.gov/nchs/products/databriefs/db127.htm.

16 Gillin, J C, C L Spinweber, and L C Johnson. "Rebound Insomnia: a Critical Review." Journal of Clinical Psychopharmacology. U.S. National Library of Medicine, June 1989. https://www.ncbi.nlm.nih.gov/pubmed/2567741.

17 Harvard Health Publishing. "The Savvy Sleeper: Wean Yourself off Sleep Aids." Harvard Health, December 2013. https://www.health.harvard.edu/staying-healthy/the-savvy-sleeper-wean-yourself-off-sleep-aids.

ACKNOWLEDGMENTS

Wow, this book has been such an adventure!

It all started when Jill Avey, enthusiastic about a sleep workshop I had facilitated at the International Coaching Federation of Washington, sent me an email one night and suggested that I write a book on the hidden powers of sleep. Jill, I didn't sleep that night! It had never occurred to me that I could reach and help more people this way. It had also never occurred to me that I had enough knowledge and experience to write a book that could impact others. Thank you for your trust in my ability to share my passion. Without you, there would be no book. Now that it's here, I hope it will be a good resource for you and the CEOs you support.

I honestly had no clue what I was getting into when I started writing this book. Even though I have loved the process and the personal growth attached to it, it has been an emotional roller coaster and a pretty high source of stress at times. Without Fabrice, my discreet but unwavering husband, this project would never have been completed. Mon Chéri, your support matters so much to me. You have no idea how influential you have been in this project, and in my life in general. My words cannot thank you enough.

A huge thank you also to my three daughters, Lola, Salomé, and Elisa. Elisa, you have always been able to cheer me up when I was discouraged. You have been very generous with this talent of yours. Also, your great cooking provided me with the fuel I needed to think straight and work long hours. Thank you, sweetheart! Salomé, there were tasks along the way that got me completely stuck. I had no clue how to give my book visual softness. You came up with beautiful illustrations, and when I was overwhelmed just thinking about writing a reference list, you took the project off my hands. It was that simple! Thank you for bringing solutions when I saw problems. Lola, you were my very first editor and found a way to turn my rambling into clear and concise writing. My initial draft was quite a mess, but you rolled up your sleeves and, thanks to your patience and great writing skills, you turned it into an inspiring and motivational tool that I was proud to send to Celia Speirs, my highly efficient, dependable, and thoughtful copy-editor.

I could never have done this without tremendous help from a few special people. Renee LeBoeuf, Elise Kloter, Christine Suter, and Holli Margel, not only did you take hours of your time to read my manuscript and give me your honest and constructive feedback, but you also provided the encouragement I needed to keep working and bring this book to the next level. I am extremely grateful for what you have done for me and I can assure you that at no point did I take any of your work and comments for granted.

Keith Creighton, you gave me a space and beautiful words to talk about my own life and sleep. Jeff Keller, you gave me a ride when I most needed it; Kanchan Shindlauer, you trusted me enough to share my work with others and as a result made my world bigger and brighter. Thank you all; I feel very lucky that our paths have crossed.

Thank you to the friends and relatives who believed in me and supported me all along. Freddie Fiorani-Campbell, Gwen Sauvage, and Nadia Loichot, the press articles you sent me regularly not only helped me in my work but also showed me that you cared. Aida Lynch, Behnaz Mansouri, Jana Claxton, Sophie Laurent-Hallet, Tara Cowe-Spigai, and Tricia DiBernardo-Thomas, you believed in me, and I knew all along that I could count on your support. Merci!

Many thanks to all the contributors to this book. Nancy Ishii, Mary Torres, Anthony Gitch, Tamara Gillest, and Christopher Hill, you have greatly enhanced the value of my book and made it richer with tangible tips that, I am sure, my dear readers will appreciate.

Thank you to all my amazing Advance Readers. You were a dream team and your enthusiasm for this book has given me wings.

I am also very grateful to the researchers, authors, podcasters, influencers, and journalists who work tirelessly to share their knowledge about sleep, and who understand how important it is to be well-rested. They are actively making the world a better place, and their studies, books, shows, and articles were invaluable resources as I was doing research to write this book.

Finally, I am extremely grateful to all the people who, every day, make my job possible. My dear clients, and you, dedicated reader. Without your trust, I wouldn't be able to exercise my passion day in and day out, and I wouldn't have collected all the "STORYTIME" inserts and the real-life situations presented in this book. Thank you for sharing your experiences and struggles with me. Thank you for taking the time to be part of my journey and letting me be part of yours. Thank you beyond words to all of you.

ABOUT THE AUTHOR

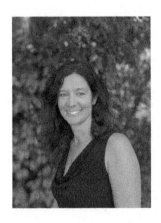

Born and raised in France where she spent the first 30 years of her life, Stella Loichot discovered the power of healthy living long before moving to the United States and settling in beautiful Seattle, where she now thrives with her husband and three daughters.

Witnessing the struggle many adults experience when trying to reconcile a healthy lifestyle with a fun and enjoyable life, she decided to focus her energy on simplifying the process for them and leading them to life-changing success.

Certified by the National Board for Health and Wellness Coaching (NBHWC) and trained in myriad modalities such as Behavioral Change, Motivational Interviewing, Weight Management and Diabetes Prevention Coaching, and Small Group Facilitation, she has a special love of working with those affected by prediabetes, a condition relevant to more than 1 in 3 adults in the US and anticipated to reach over 8% of the global adult population by 2045.

To discuss coaching, speaking, and corporate wellness opportunities, please contact Stella directly.

Stella Loichot, NBC-HWC
stella@allonzcoaching.com
allonZcoaching.com/contact/

Made in the USA
Coppell, TX
30 October 2020